Trust in Experience

Transferable learning for primary care trusts

Edited by
Geoff Meads and Tricia Meads

Foreword by
Professor Mike Pringle

Radcliffe Medical Press

Radcliffe Medical Press Ltd
18 Marcham Road, Abingdon, Oxon OX14 1AA

British Library Cataloguing in Publication Data

A catalogue record for this book is available from the British Library.

ISBN 1 85775 457 3

Typeset by Aarontype Ltd, Easton, Bristol
Printed and bound TJ International Ltd, Padstow, Cornwall

The writing of this book has been supported by an Eli Lilly research grant.

Contents

Foreword

Many, myself included, saw the election of a new Labour administration in 1997 as a watershed for general practice and primary care. I expected the demolition of fundholding to presage a swing of the pendulum from the rhetoric of a 'primary care led-NHS' towards either a 'management-led NHS' or a 'hospital-led NHS'. There were genuine fears that we had had our chance in the sunshine and that we were about to enter the umbra of diminished importance.

Some have not yet realised still the error in this analysis. The focus of influence has changed but primary care's position has been strengthened. The practice is no longer pre-eminent, but it has not been replaced by a reformed 'FHSA'. We now have community level organisations – primary care groups and trusts – that have reinvented the primary care centre of the NHS in England.

While fundholding practices developed influence and skills that they applied for their own patients, their commitment to a wider local health community was often weak. Under PCTs, the strength of individual practices and their primary care teams has been diluted. Indeed, it can be argued that the power of individual general practitioners and of the general practitioner community has been reduced. For some this is a source of regret; for others it is the empowering of all primary care disciplines.

In a world in which variations in care – especially under-performance – are no longer acceptable and in which standards must be locally delivered, the practice increasingly looks like the right unit to deliver care, but not to commission or manage it. In the smaller PCTs the population size is at the lower limits of efficiency for commissioning for populations and yet the largest are still able to reflect the characteristics of their population.

If standards of care in primary care and service configurations throughout the NHS lie in the hands of these new bodies, we must consider their competency for this task. Some of their skills have come from health authorities, some from fundholding and some from community trusts. Considering the scope for cultural conflict between these backgrounds, PCTs have made a remarkable start in establishing themselves.

However, these skills alone will not be sufficient. Fundholding staff can provide 'general practice' and 'commissioning' perspectives; health authority staff can offer 'organisation' and 'management' skills; those from community trust backgrounds can offer multidisciplinary and human resource skills – but PCTs will need more.

They will need political, systems engineering and strategic skills. They must deliver on quality assurance, service development and benchmarking. Their leadership will extend into consultations and clinical decisions throughout their area in order to get quality care – National Service Frameworks, NICE guidelines, best practice – available to every patient. And they must monitor the care of their populations, matching health need to service development in order to reduce inequalities and improve outcomes.

This is not a trivial agenda! Indeed, it is arguably the most demanding list of expectations ever placed on health service organisations in England. And these are nascent PCTs, starved of management cash and with an uncertain pedigree. Under these circumstances PCTs need to learn all they can from each other's experience. They need to avoid reinventing successes and replicating errors.

This readable and informative book sets out and succeeds in offering a paradigm for the transfer of experience. It is an essential read for every person involved in PCTs in England, and in similar organisations throughout the UK. Those coming to terms with the new NHS need to understand the networking and sharing potential that lies within the experience of all PCTs today – a potential that is explored between these covers.

Professor Mike Pringle
Chairman of Council
Royal College of General Practitioners
January 2001

Preface

We can bridge the gulf between the reality of the NHS today and the vision of what it should be like tomorrow.[1]

This book represents another kind of third way. In seeking to strengthen those involved with the development of NHS primary care trusts, it offers an alternative source of assistance to either national policy guidance on the one hand (*see* Appendix 1) or individual management consultants' expertise on the other (e.g. Lilley 2000). Arguably, the New NHS, partly as a result of possessing this very title, has already witnessed enough of both. The wheel can only be reinvented so many times. Our third way tries to recognise this. The chapters that follow are, therefore, not about 'new' learning but about the application of existing knowledge. The aim is to help generate a real commitment to the new organisations by enabling their participants to make practical use of: relevant past and parallel NHS experience; comparable developments in other public services and sometimes other countries; the appropriate research literature; and the almost inexhaustible range of working models and concepts these can supply.

This sense of commitment has often been lacking, in our experience, over the past two years. Feelings of actual ownership have not yet embraced many of the new primary care organisations at the end of 2000. They remain essentially a central creature and the freelance facilitator's paradise. There are many well rehearsed reasons for this general ennui. The practical burden of shifting from the pre-1997 internal market into a social system *modus operandi* has been heavy. It has been hard to see the wood for the trees. Organisational instability and uncertainty has been pervasive throughout the New NHS. Unlike in previous times there have been no fixed points in the healthcare environment serving as the pivotal change agents for others. Even in primary care, many have felt the basic practice unit threatened by the advent of such potential alternatives as walk-in centres and telephone helplines; and the future prospects of partner health authorities and NHS community trusts, in particular, seem precarious. Over 3000 GP fundholding units have been abolished. People, and professionals especially, have had to adjust to the reassertion of political leadership and administration with a plethora of revised arrangements for their probity and public accountability.

---

[1] *NHS Plan* 2000: 1.29

Clinical governance, the NHS Plan, National Service Frameworks and the new czars are simply the most publicised examples of this new, apparently all-pervasive context.

In circumstances such as these it is hard to believe decentralisation really is taking place. NHS primary care trusts can all too easily be regarded as an imposition rather than an opportunity and, curiously, the harder central civil servants try to clarify the scope of the new organisations through more circulars and conferences, the worse it often actually seems to feel. The space for experimentation, for trial and error, for getting things down-right wrong, becomes ever more limited. And all of these are the essential ingredients of making something your own. So far, too few care too little about primary care trusts. Significantly, over three years into the post-fund-holding period it remains difficult in primary care to name local champions of the cause. The popular platform speakers are still few and far between. The heroic tradition of individual GP-based primary care in the UK appears to be coming to an end.

In part, this is because thinking, and speaking, independently in respect of the contemporary NHS has become seen as, at best, unfashionable and at worst unacceptable. You are either onside with NHS primary care trusts and their associated reforms, or you are not. And if you are not then you have to find another game. This perception is a pity. Questioning, at all levels, helps to gain the kind of commitment Drucker refers to below as becoming the critical component of future citizenship and contemporary public services:

> Every developed country needs an autonomous, self-governing social sector of community organisations. It needs it to provide the needed community services. It needs it above all to provide the bonds of community and to restore active citizenship. Historically community was fate. In the post-capitalist society and polity community has to become commitment. (Drucker 1994: p. 161)

It is through the answers we find to our questions that we move into real relationships with the New NHS. Primary care trusts can turn in this process from organisational hosts to organisational homes. And if the answers have the robust quality of independent appraisal then the strength of the commitment can reflect this rigour. The writers in this book have been charged with delivering defensible independent appraisals in their specific subject area. Each of the latter has been selected for its utilitarian purpose. Together they constitute the critical interfaces where primary care trusts will stand or fall as organisations: with social services; with public health and the new NHS mental health trusts; with regulators and agents of financial control; with managed care and hospitals of all types; and with a patient public itself. In each case the writer of the designated chapter has not sought to critique government policy. Embarrassing the Secretary of State is not part of the brief. On the contrary, indeed, all of the contributors support the overall central policy direction. Their contribution is to enhance this by making available as applied academics the kinds of evidence and experience that, in the form of independent appraisals, may be most akin to the needs of those in primary care where the culture of independence itself has conventionally been at its most deep-rooted. Historically, GPs, dentists, optometrists and other family health services professionals have reacted rather than responded to central policy direction. Many of their most enduring developments owe their origins to the independent status of primary care practitioners. This book is true to this tradition.

Its contributors are mostly drawn from the staff and their associates in the Health Management Group of City University. From its central London base, they have worked, over the past three years, with almost half of the original 481 primary care groups. It is a unique, nationwide pool of experience, based, unlike that of other universities, on a wide variety of sponsors, with little direct government support through, for example, mainstream NHS research and development contracts. This multi-funding, ranging from life sciences companies to the Bible Society, facilitates an independent perspective. We are not beholden to anybody. The writers can state freely what works and what does not and, as a result, what could be either usable or useless.

The Health Management Group currently offers four postgraduate degree-level teaching programmes and some of the material in the book has been taken into these, sometimes through teaching in seminars and simulations, and sometimes as subject matter for project-based enquiry and dissertations. The chapters by Benaim, Berridge and Cohen, for example, each have their origins in the MSc in Contemporary Health and Social Policy, while both Barker and Tucker have been registered for MPhil degrees. These students are in the guise of either associate researchers or lecturer-practitioners and several of the HMG staff also have this 'boundroiduality' that the King's Fund and other applied research institutes seem to find so valuable in the NHS development work (Poxton 1999: pp. 1–3). The chapters on the benefits of 'new partnerships' and 'transferable learning' by Ashcroft and Geoff Meads respectively, for example, owe a great deal to the writers' combined roles in a series of recent collaborative ventures between the Health Management Group and the Cambridge-based Relationships Foundation. Individual health districts have served as the principal data sources for the material on managed care, managing change and financial management contained in the chapters prepared by Hill and Hudson, Tricia Meads and Moore, while both regional surveys and national pilot sites have fed into the research of Coleman, Cornish and Petchey. All of these look to learning beyond local boundaries, and the application of concepts and ideas from outside the NHS, past and present, is best demonstrated in the models of decision making, scenario planning and participation described in the contributions by Cramp, Geoff Meads and Winkler. Collectively the individual papers are a rich resource. Together they suggest that while the New NHS as a corporate identity can claim to be genuinely novel, nothing in its component parts is really new. Everything has a reference point. There is no need to feel out of your depth. In these interesting times it is a reassuring message. It means that NHS primary care trusts can live up to their name.

The book is set out in three sections. The first, entitled 'Policy into Practice', takes the translation of central policy statements into local operational practice as its basic premise. There are three chapters in this section, prepared by the book's editors. The first explores what might be termed the text's thematic of *transferable learning*, and how this can be applied widely and imaginatively to new NHS primary care trusts. The second is derived directly from the juxtaposition between national guidance and local experience, with much of the material drawn from this project's specific PCG/T sites and the interviews with the individual executive officers who kindly accepted the invitation to contribute to this publication. The focus here is on the tensions they have encountered seeking to bridge the space between policy and practice, and on the transferable learning they have both sought and still need to resolve these tensions. Clinical improvement, relationships management and local alliances emerge as three important targets for this learning. The third chapter looks again at how rhetoric and realities can be reconciled by PCTs, this time through robust resource utilisation criteria and frameworks drawn from recent fieldwork experience and expertise, and the application of robust professional accountancy principles.

The second section reverses the relationship between the central and local boundaries of the NHS, but sustains the thematic of transferable learning. A series of 11 working papers comprehensively addresses the actual tasks involved in turning primary care organisations into objects of trust. The focus and title here is 'Practice into Policy'. The purpose is to point to how NHS primary care trusts can themselves take the leading role in creating the national policy of which they have so far been simply the subject.

The short, final, section, by Derek Cramp, the HMG Professor of Health Systems, Fedelma Winkler and Geoff Meads, is a synthesis designed to respond to its title 'Looking Ahead'. It brings together specific lessons from the separate contributors into a single set of future scenarios and recommendations in the context of the 2000 NHS National Plan. In particular, it addresses the vital issue of why and how primary care trusts should look to help restore the credibility of a national health service. The target readership is those responsible for creating the locally viable new primary care organisations which may evolve into viable future Care Trusts. This aspiration becomes achievable if the target readership means not simply PCT board members but all those at primary care fieldwork level who want to be part of an NHS in the future that can be taken on trust.

The editors would like to express their appreciation to all those who have participated in the preparation of this book. They include not just the chapter contributors, but the PCG/T chief executives who agreed to take part in individual interviews; the primary care groups in Bridgwater, Croydon, Hythe, Islington, Harrogate and elsewhere that hosted HMG workshops during the specific period of the book's preparation; and to all the other primary care organisations that have participated in our associated research. There are simply too many to mention here by name (*see* Appendix 2).

Finally, special thanks are due in two directions. First, Eli Lilly for both co-sponsoring the project and providing its NHS Diabetic Services Manager, Roger Hudson, to the project team in what is no doubt a sign of future times for primary care trusts. Second, thanks go to Moira Dustin and Charlotte Parry, our research assistant and administrator, respectively, to whom credit for any coherence that emerges from such a complex and complicated project is due.

This book is dedicated to our children.

Geoff and Tricia Meads
January 2001

References

NHSE (1999) *Primary Care Trusts: establishment, the preparatory period and their functions.* Department of Health, London.

Drucker P (1994) *Post-Capitalist Society.* Butterworth-Heinemann, Oxford.

Lilley R (2000) *The Primary Care Trust Tool Kit.* Radcliffe Medical Press, Oxford.

Poxton R (ed) (1999) *Working Across the Boundaries.* King's Fund, London.

List of contributors

John Ashcroft is Research Director of the Relationships Foundation at the Jubilee Centre, Cambridge where he manages the Relational Health Care Project in a collaborative venture with the HMG.

Jacqui Barker is a Fellow in Organisational Development at the Office for Public Management, an HMG postgraduate researcher and former Assistant Director of Public Health Commissioning for Bromley Health Authority.

Rosie Benaim is Research Officer for the Camden Blind People's Association and an associate researcher for the HMG and King's Fund.

Michael Berridge is a GP and PCG member in Leeds, and a former HMG postgraduate research student.

Elaine Cohen is Director of Primary Care for Marylebone PCG and an HMG postgraduate research student.

David Coleman is a community pharmacist and PCG prescribing adviser in Sussex and Hampshire, with research interests at City and Portsmouth Universities.

Yvonne Cornish is a Lecturer in Health Policy with Kent and City Universities and an HMG researcher.

Derek Cramp holds Visiting Professorships in Medical Systems and Health Management with City and Surrey Universities and is an HMG researcher.

Marie Hill is a practice nurse and PCG nurse adviser in Lambeth, Southwark and Lewisham health district, and a former HMG postgraduate research student. She is currently on a one-year secondment as Lecturer in Community and Primary Care Nursing, St Bartholomew's School of Nursing & Midwifery.

Roger Hudson is Diabetic Services Manager for Eli Lilly Industries Ltd.

Geoff Meads is HMG Professor of Health Services Development at City University, and formerly an NHS regional director.

Tricia Meads is a Finance Manager for Southampton and South West Hampshire, and an HMG occasional Lecturer on Primary Care Finance.

Robert Moore is Head of Health Development for North Peterborough PCT, and a former HMG postgraduate research student.

Roland Petchey is HMG Director and PCG/PMS Research Programmes Co-ordinator.

Mike Pringle is a GP in Nottingham, Professor of General Practice at the Queen's Medical Centre and Chairman of the RCGP Council.

Helen Tucker is Chair of the Community Hospitals Association for England and Wales, a management consultant and HMG researcher.

Leroy White is Reader in Public Health Policy at South Bank University in London.

Fedelma Winkler is an HMG Visiting Lecturer in Primary Care Development and a former FHSA and CHC chief officer.

List of abbreviations

AAA	Annual Accountability Agreement
A&E	Accident and Emergency
CEE	Clinical Effectiveness Evidence
CHA	Community Hospitals Association
CHD	Coronary Heart Disease
CIPFA	Chartered Institute of Public Finance Accountancy
CPD	Continuing Professional Development
DCFS	Directorate of Counter Fraud Services
DGH	District General Hospital
DHA	District Health Authority
DoH	Department of Health
DPC	District Prescribing Committee
DPH	Director of Public Health
DTI	Department of Trade and Industry
EBM	Evidence-Based Medicine
EC	Executive Committee
FHS	Family Health Services
FHSA	Family Health Services Authority
FPHM	Faculty of Public Health Medicine
GDP	Gross Domestic Product
GMC	General Medical Council
GMS	General Medical Services
GP	General Practitioner
GPC	General Practice Committee
GPFH	General Practice Fundholding
GUT	Grand Unifying Theory
HA	Health Authority
H&HSR	Health and Health Services Research
HAZ	Health Action Zone
HCHS	Hospitals and Community Health Services
HFA	Health for All
HImP	Health Improvement Programme
HMG	Health Management Group
HMSO	Her Majesty's Stationery Office
HNA	Health Needs Assessment
ICP	Integrated Care Pathways
IM&T	Information Management and Technology
ISO	International Standards Organisation
IT	Information Technology

KCW	Kensington, Chelsea and Westminster
LA	Local Authority
LIS	Local Implementation Strategy
LMC	Local Medical Committee
MAAG	Medical Audit Advisory Group
MBO	Management by Objectives
MDS	Minimum Data Set
NHS	National Health Service
NICE	National Institute for Clinical Excellence
NPC	National Prescribing Centre
NSF	National Service Framework
OAT	Out-of-Area Treatment
OD	Organisational Development
ONS	Office of National Statistics
OTC	Over-the-counter
PACE	Promoting Action on Clinical Effectiveness
PACT	Prescribing Analysis and Cost
PCG	Primary Care Group
PCIP	Primary Care Investment Plan
PCT	Primary Care Trust
PDP	Personal Development Plan
PFI	Private Finance Initiative
PHCT	Primary Healthcare Team
PMS	Personal Medical Services
PPA	Prescription Pricing Authority
PPP	Public–Private Partnership
PPRS	Prescription Price Regulation Scheme
PRIMIS	Primary Care Information Services
PSP	Practice Support Pharmacist
RAWP	Research Allocation Working Party
R&D	Research and Development
RCT	Randomised Control Trial
RCGP	Royal College of General Practitioners
RF	Relationships Foundation
RPSGB	Royal Pharmaceutical Society of Great Britain
SaFF	Service and Financial Framework
SIFTR	Service Increment for Teaching and Research
SLA	Service Level Agreement
SSD	Social Services Department
TARGET	Time for Audit, Review, Guidelines, Education and Training
TPP	Total Purchasing Project
TQM	Total Quality Management
UK	United Kingdom
VFM	Value For Money
WHO	World Health Organization

To
Sarah, Matthew and Rebecca

Those who can be trusted will be given more

Matthew 25:29

PART 1

Policy into practice

Geoff Meads and Tricia Meads

CHAPTER 1

Transferable learning

The NHS continues to work at the cutting edge of new forms of health services.[1]

Tensions

That it should be in a state of tension with local practice, and that this tension should be a creative force, is an essential characteristic of central policy and its effective development. Sometimes this means harnessing the energy of disparate individual initiatives, which have been self-generated, and converting them into a national pattern – as if this were what was intended all along. Such was the case, for example, in October 1994, when total purchasing pilots and community fundholding were introduced ostensibly as extensions to the existing standard GP fundholding scheme (GPFH), thereby assuming control of a range of local organisational developments sponsored by health commissions and regional health authorities. And just for good measure, to complete the 'colonisation' effect both of the latter were swiftly abolished and most of their functions transferred to the Department of Health's own regional offices.

On the other hand, sometimes the creative tension arises when central policy needs genuinely to set the agenda. Such is the case with NHS primary care trusts (PCTs). They are unequivocally a central creature. Of course, they can be depicted as a linear progression from a historic perspective, and Figure 1.1 illustrates the parallel shifts from independent family health services practitioners to corporate primary care organisation, and from individual patient to a community population, that have characterised the overall changes in formal relationships over the last decade. The new trusts are, however, much better understood from a lateral than a vertical perspective. They make more sense in the context of political devolution; of international developments in managed care and primary health services; and in relation to contemporary models of complex organisations, which no longer respect separate sectoral and professional

---

[1] *NHS Plan* 2000: 2.4

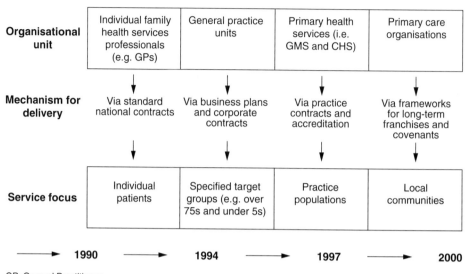

Organisational unit	Individual family health services professionals (e.g. GPs)	General practice units	Primary health services (i.e. GMS and CHS)	Primary care organisations
Mechanism for delivery	Via standard national contracts	Via business plans and corporate contracts	Via practice contracts and accreditation	Via frameworks for long-term franchises and covenants
Service focus	Individual patients	Specified target groups (e.g. over 75s and under 5s)	Practice populations	Local communities
	1990	1994	1997	2000

GP: General Practitioner
GMS: General Medical Services
CHS: Community Health Services

Figure 1.1   Contemporary primary care development. *Source*: Meads 1999: p. 23.

boundaries in their pursuit of optimal resource investment. The energies that central policy are seeking to harness and control in NHS PCTs are, accordingly, not so much those of local entrepreneurs, at local practice level, but those of newly elected assembly representatives with public service mandates and expenditure powers; of care agencies right across the spectrum of ownership and their sponsors; and of those 'virtual' and 'stakeholder' enterprises which at macroeconomic levels are critically important to the future design of any public service system. The life science company, the centrally designated development zone, and progressive anti-monopoly legislation at European Union levels, for example, represent the world into which NHS PCTs must fit.

NHS PCTs will not simply slip into this scenario by a process of natural evolution. It is the responsibility of central policy to determine the direction. New primary care organisations must be subjected to the pressures required for their accelerated development.

For those working in primary care, this modern policy formulation role remains difficult to understand and even harder to accept. The NHS as a whole is still an insular institution. Early local studies of PCGs confirm a 'lack of awareness of the wider environment' (Eve and Mares 2000) and the vital 'importance of developing learning processes in new organisations' (Wilkin *et al.* 2000). The NHS is not good at transferable learning. Within its boundaries, the family health services professionals, and general medical and dental practitioners in particular, are usually proud of their independent employment status. Unfortunately this pride has too often translated itself into horizons which do not scan far beyond the surgery or local health centre. Through these eyes, the PCT is perceived simply as another phase in the continuous organisational transition of the NHS. It merely represents a successor body to the executive councils, family practitioner committees and family health services authorities, with elements of the traditional local representative committee thrown in for good measure to keep the professions, and in particular the doctors, sweet and onside. In its limitations this is a dangerously partial perspective. It creates the illusion that the new PCTs are a passing phenomenon. It undermines their meaning and reduces that creative tension which should exist between policy and practice.

This tension is, of course, an intrinsic part of the reciprocal relationship between those sited at the two central and local boundaries of the NHS. It is here that political power is exerted: by ministers with a parliamentary constituency of citizens' votes, and GPs with a professional constituency of seemingly insatiable consumer demand. On a bad day, in winter, this may consist of as many as a million consultations a day. Both political bases are strong and enduring. The relationships between them in the past have often been characterised by a scale of tension that has escalated into outright conflicts. Remarkably, several of these, in terms of primary care development, have proved both highly creative and useful. The germ of the group practice was the £800 000 development fund left over in 1951, following a long-running remuneration dispute which dated back to the final days of the Second World War. The GP Charter in 1966 that, for the first time, created through central policy the funded local employment infrastructures for practice team development, followed the serious threat of mass resignations from the NHS two years earlier. And, in the closing phase of the last century, chronic disease management rose as a systematic feature of primary care provision from the ashes of abortive attempts to establish health promotion clinics in every general practice, through the terms of the 1990 General Medical Services Contract.

Despite these benefits, or indeed because of the ways in which they have been achieved, a combative culture has been created for and between government and general practice. It is one in which the decentralisation represented by the advent of PCTs is automatically treated with suspicion, even though it represents a completely unprecedented level of resource management responsibilities transferred to local settings. PCTs, at level 4, will typically manage around 80% of the NHS funds allocated for their local population, through their commissioning functions. In many instances this will exceed £100 million. At face value, it is an extraordinary development. But those who are the recipients of what the Minister for Health described as 'a range of freedoms and flexibilities not currently available to any other health service body' (Denham 1999) are wary. Does this decentralisation truly signify liberation and licence; or is it about incorporating general practice within a politically controlled, performance-managed institution? On a daily basis will it prevent the GP advocating on behalf of patients for relief from the social and economic conditions that cause illness by becoming part of the political decision-making processes that contribute to the creation of these conditions? (Heath 1995: pp. 42–43). In short, centrally-imposed decentralisation can seem like a contradiction in terms. National policy is top-down and primary care development should be, aetiologically, bottom-up.

Trust

This legacy of suspicion, combined with the partial understanding of the broader context and sources of the new primary care organisations, leads to the paradoxical position of the new NHS trusts being regarded fundamentally with mistrust. For many practitioners their title belies their truth, for *trust* in central policy is seen as a distant relation to its counterpart in local practice. The term, in the NHS, has four significant connotations: organisational, quasi-legal, professional and ethical. At one end of the policy spectrum, the value of *trust* as a policy concept is the solid meaning it conveys publicly to communities and their representatives about new models of service provision. At the other end of this spectrum, the term *trust* is also at the heart of the confidential encounter between vulnerable, sick and infirm individuals and their carers. The problem arises when, by design or default, meanings are transferred: when professional relationships are politicised, or when policy definitions – such as that of the *primary care-led NHS* – are made so malleable as to lack intellectual integrity and worth.

In this respect 1991 and 2001 represent a curious juxtaposition. When NHS trusts were introduced to secondary care in 1991 the concern was that their freedoms were excessive and their public accountabilities insufficient. As the first major wave of PCTs prepares for its April 2001 launch, the concerns are that basically the same regime represents what one PCG chief executive described to us as 'the threat to our powers of self-determination'.

The organisational and quasi-legal connotations of *trust* are mutually reinforcing. Together they have a respectable ring. The solicitor may understand the term as:

> Coming about as a result of a decision on the part of both the settler and the trustee that it should... (Gardner 1990: p. 5)

It is authoritatively defined as:

> An equitable obligation which binds a person to deal with some
> specific property for the benefit of the persons or the advance-
> ment of some specific purpose. (Ford 1974: p. 1)

This is the basis for contracts and covenants, for the leaving of legacies
and the giving of grants. It presupposes reciprocity and consent. Like all
attractive contemporary policy concepts – *quality* and *equity* are the most
obvious others – *trust* has multiple meanings. As such it can convey a sense
of the profound, as in the universal truths of a parable; or conversely it can
communicate at the level of the lowest common denominator. Employed
this way, *trust* has all the superficial attractions of an advertising slogan; and
little else to commend its usage.

Hence the concerns in its application to primary care, in the settings
of which the ethics of professional and personal relationships have to be
paramount. If these are endangered then, as Starfield (1992: p. 7) has noted
the 'philosophical underpinnings' of the whole health and healthcare system
are placed in jeopardy. At this level the term signifies a secure confidence
between two partners, a certain faith and a sound basis for change; even
for taking risks and sharing in the anticipated experience of unknown and
dangerous conditions. For those working in primary care, trust as such
is a precious principle. Its projection onto the quasi-legal organisational
framework of the new NHS PCTs devalues its worth. Far from supply-
ing reassurance, it disturbs. The importance of the new organisations living
up to their name could scarcely, therefore, be overstated. They need to
be genuinely about primary care; and we need to be able to take this
on trust.

Understanding the different creative tensions required for central policy
development and for local primary care development, and the inevitable
further differences arising from their increased interaction as a result of
the advent of the new PCTs, helps to promote understanding and
tolerance. The common NHS rituals of simplistic scapegoating by one side
of the other and traditional stereotyping are even less acceptable in this
context. NHS PCTs as complex systems occupy what some contemporary
GP researchers have called 'phase space' in which both actual and potential future courses of development are understood as occupants; and
minor adjustments can lead to major changes in the system (Griffiths
and Byrne 1998).

Accordingly, these new organisations are better assessed through, for
example, scenario planning, simulations and cluster or critical path analyses,
than through traditional positivist research methods focused largely on the
clinical discipline of general medical practice.

As Chapter 15 argues, such a focus is now clearly far too narrow. There is a pressing need to apply to PCTs the principle of transferable learning from across the NHS; from allied health and healthcare systems elsewhere; from comparable organisational developments in housing, education and the other public services; and educationally from the theoretical models and applied concepts of the relevant research literature. Otherwise, NHS PCTs will continue to be seen as completely new, a 'one-off'; a unique product of 'modernisation'; and a mystery and mystique will surround them. This would not be helpful. General practice has suffered from the illusion of being more than it was, with excessive expectations as an ever-growing consequence. It is important not to make the same mistake with PCTs.

Actually, given the scale of their new responsibilities, it is absolutely vital that they do not follow into the same trap. Their basic responsibilities have been defined by central policy as virtually synonymous with the purpose of the NHS itself: promoting public health, commissioning effective secondary care and integrating primary health services into community care (Secretary of State 1997: p. 34). That PCTs are intended to be the local voice of the NHS was crystal clear in the Minister of Health's personal letter to all NHS board members of the 19 February 1999 (Denham 1999). This defines the trusts' five critical relationships with: practices, individual clinicians, community services, patients and local providers. In each case, closer proximity is the goal, through better support, access and participation. On each count the NHS institution has historically scored low, usually being characterised by the features of an essentially medical model, a paternalistic culture and the autonomy of specialists. PCTs have a lot to learn and much of what they have to learn is not available from the NHS, either past or present. In a profound sense their future depends on discovering a new sense of trust in others, many of whom are newcomers, foreigners and strangers.

Transnationalism

Transferable learning is the theme of this book, and globalisation is the first theme of the so-called 'Third Way' (Giddens 1998). In the chapters that follow, most of the learning on offer comes either from settings parallel to the NHS in the UK, or from different parts of the NHS itself. Globalisation looks to the macro-forces of international economic structures; borderless networks of information exchange and technological development; and increasingly influential global policy sources, as major determinants of how national organisations are shaped. The developing countries of, for example, Central America or the former communist states of Eastern

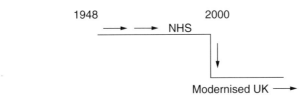

Figure 1.2   Catastrophe cliff.

Europe with growing gross domestic products (GDPs) allied to a degree of external sponsorship and instruction, through such agencies as the World Bank and World Health Organization, are particularly susceptible to these global forces. Accordingly, they represent an especially rich source of learning for the UK, and particularly those in primary care, now that the permanence of the general practice unit can no longer be assumed. We are having to recognise in our 'modernised' new NHS that we can no longer shut out the outside world. The scenario of the catastrophe cliff outlined in Figure 1.2 is all too readily recognisable. Transferable learning is at its most valuable when it is not just interesting but also clearly applicable; preferably with a sharp edge to it as well.

Two simple illustrations provide evidence to support the principle of 'globalisation' and its transferable learning. Costa Rica and Moldova may seem unlikely sources and resources. No doubt there will be some readers who will not be quite sure where to find them in the atlas. It would be hard, however, to conclude that at least some of their features should not be found in the future on our NHS map. Selected for their obscurity, the sense of apparent irrelevance quickly turns to one of potential utility as their particular organisational models are explored. The truth is that a complacent conservative community sector in the UK has much to learn from almost anywhere.

The pivotal unit of much primary care in Costa Rica is the *ebais*. In a part of the world only recently emerging from a succession of military dictatorships, the *ebais* is part of the elected government's attempt to forge a new relationship with its people. Deceptively simple in style and substance, the *ebais* is a local clinic with half a dozen rooms and usually about the same number of staff. These usually comprise a doctor (with five or six years' training), a primary care nurse practitioner, three health technicians, plus sessional inputs from community pharmacists, opticians and other welfare workers. Each *ebais* covers a population of 8000 people. Each day the health technicians undertake a minimum of eight domiciliary visits. Supervised by the nurse, and with direct access to the doctor, they target both those who are priorities for intervention – particularly in terms of illness prevention – and compile simple but comprehensive health and social needs profiles in a standard computerised format. Every household must be visited each year.

Through the national networks the aggregated information is automatically available at every level: at the *ebais* to determine individual care and treatment priorities; at the provincial hospitals to shape service developments; and nationally to steer public health strategies and clinical education programmes. The *ebais*, the provincial centres and the university teaching hospital in the capital, San José, are all electronically linked.

Telemedicine means that expert consultation is rapidly accessed from even the remotest areas, and training inputs are available regularly throughout the 24-hour day. It is impressive and relatively cheap. The health technicians receive six months' training. A constant theme throughout the developing countries of Central America is the economic and social necessity of avoiding the 'professional capture' which so characterises healthcare organisations and their services in the so-called developed 'First World', of which the UK is a core member.

Costa Rica has used the Internet well, both to shape its own primary care system and to learn the pitfalls and potential of others. It has been selective. Those responsible for its design quote a disarming range of sources. The health technician's role is derived from the approach of non-governmental organisations across the Indian subcontinent. The use of new information technology techniques is taken from the commercial, managed care enterprises of the eastern United States. The use of public taxation and comprehensive state insurance arrangements refer to the United Kingdom, Taiwan and Holland; and the British experience curiously is also mentioned in relation to successful models of provider deregulation and market management. The proactive role of the State in assuming a direct and indeed controlling responsibility for the health status of the national community as a whole copies Cuba. This approach is nothing if not eclectic.

Of course, however, such an 'ideal type' initiative as that in Costa Rica will not endure unless there is a cultural fit. The early months of 2000 did witness typically noisy street demonstrations against some elements of the healthcare reforms. Opening up provider agencies to private ownership, including some of the *ebais*, is not popular with some of the trade unions. Nevertheless, that there are elements of transferable learning is obvious. Moreover, this is evident at all levels, from the way in which central policy and its principles are developed, to the daily details of operational service delivery. Health Action Zones and Healthy Living Centres, let alone the new PCTs, could certainly learn a thing or two.

Not surprisingly, contemporary primary care in the 40 medical directorates that make up the geographic *raion* of Moldova has a rather different list of references. If the skills of 'political spin', UK-style, had been learnt in this small landlocked country to the west of the Black Sea, then it could describe itself as having taken the best bits from its Russian inheritance, while at the same time learning to align itself with its new Balkan neighbours – who themselves have drawn heavily in several instances on material from China. Stripped of the political spin, the truth in practice is rather more mundane. The realities of Moldova are a curious ethnic mix of peoples with Romanian, Russian and Ukrainian, as well as native and gypsy origins, and the country has frequently been on the verge of not one but several civil wars throughout its largely rural regions. Like Costa Rica, it is a developing country but still suffers from substantial poverty, which is as much environmental as it is economic. A polluted water bed of several metres depth is the most obvious example and, as in Costa Rica, the proportion of the national GDP spent on healthcare is declining to around 3.5% as the commercial income-generating sectors struggle for growth.

In these circumstances the pivotal unit of primary care is the village centre, the local 'medical point'. This is financed officially by the State, and less officially from other sources of the rampant black economy. The strength of the latter is indicated by the remarkable phenomenon of levels of personal taxation of over 100% and helps to explain the presence of staffing in the centres which often appears to exceed the centrally prescribed core elements of a community nurse and two doctors, with paediatric and geriatric and/or gynaecological specialist training respectively. These centres certainly do not need a 'drop-in' title; they are fundamentally community facilities. As such, they are used to host village meals, as the obvious place where a co-operative approach to basic subsistence and dietary standards can be ensured. And, of course, China-style videos on family planning or HIV prevention automatically attract large audiences in these centres as well.

It is easy to disregard such alternative primary care models on grounds of cultural difference or simply sheer ignorance. For PCTs, with the 'blank sheet' opportunities of authentically new organisations, this would be a foolish and slightly arrogant mistake. Many English primary care groups (PCGs) have stated their aspiration to be regarded as community enterprises with a generalist philosophy. Of the contributors to this book, for example, such aims have been stated publicly and explicitly by the Somerset Coast and North Islington PCGs. The Moldovan centres are actually more sophisticated than they seem. They represent the escape route from the previous multi-specialist, fee-consuming, Soviet-style polyclinics. They recognise that at the frontline the overwhelming healthcare needs are those of elderly people, female carers and the young. Their location and style mobilises a variety of forms of goods and payment, including in kind, that reduces the demands on the State purse, at a time when this is capable of subsidising no more than a few basic drugs and screening programmes. The model also, finally, gives the massive surplus of largely Moscow-trained medical personnel the chance to move into more generalist roles and to supplement their meagre official incomes through a variety of unofficial means.

On each of these four counts there is learning for an NHS PCT. This too possesses the Moldovan-style mixed organisational status of both a formal public services agency and an informal community development, making it a classic example of the modern stakeholder organisation (Meads and Ashcroft 2000: pp. 63–66). As such, it has a much wider range of resources and opportunities to draw upon than those historically available to its NHS predecessors. The creative Costa Rican developments point to just how far-reaching the scope of these might be, given imagination, goodwill and a readiness to put aside present restrictive practices and the mindsets they represent. The competitive tendency that often characterised the relationship between separate fundholding general practices has frequently applied in more recent times to the race to the line taking place between PCG chief executives. Political and performance monitoring recognition were listed by several of the latter, during our interviews, as behind the motivation to be first, and 'to be seen to be out front'. This motivation alone has been sufficient to supply the stimulus for transferable learning. All new primary care organisations should be self-generated. They need to know what is going on elsewhere to define themselves. External (good and bad) practice in an NHS where parity is still a chronic relationship issue tells an embryonic PCT where it is in the post-millennium pecking order, and where it should aim to be.

Tribalism

The sources for this learning are, therefore, as much competitive as they are collaborative. They are, accordingly, at least as well aligned with the local tensions required for primary care development as they are with the strictures of contemporary central policy guidance. Competition, of course, has conventionally been regarded as an essential element in the development of practice-based UK primary care. Each practice has been a business unit. Its income has been dependent upon attracting enough patients as customers. Each of the latter is a potential source of co-payment: sometimes small, sometimes significant. For a general medical practitioner these may amount to the fees from completing an insurance company's medical form. For a dentist a whole range of 'crowns' and cosmetic repairs means additional income, while the majority of community pharmacies today are sustained by 'over the counter' (OTC) purchases. Competing as separate suppliers for healthcare demand, and all the associated demands which can profitably be met from primary care locations, has been a key characteristic of the English family health services. Its individual professions have frequently been both commended and critiqued for their 'entrepreneurial', or even sometimes aggressive, characteristics. Moreover, the competition in primary care has been both interprofessional and intraprofessional in character. In some semi-rural areas, for example, GPs and community pharmacists both need to turn statutory supply regulations to their advantage in pursuit of monopoly rights for drugs dispensing fees. In other urban areas the independent optometrists compete with the multiple chains to offer the supplementary glaucoma and diabetic retinopathy screening programmes to the NHS that will also help guarantee a continuous stream of eyesight testing and low vision aids dispensing fees. Competition of this kind, based upon business incentives at least as much as distinctive professional expertise and education, explains why the 'old' NHS and its tribes have so often presented an easy target for policy analysts and their recommendations for radical reforms and, in some instances, actual abolition (e.g. Klein 1995; Griffiths 1996).

But 'tribalism' remains a modern necessity. Drucker terms it the necessary opposite pole to 'transnationalism' in future public service organisational development (Drucker 1994: p. 140). Integrated, multi-professional, vocationally oriented NHS PCTs can be at least as much part of this new tribalism, as they are set to become part of the new service models influenced by the kinds of global trends and influences described in the preceding section. But the tribal identity can, in future, be primary care itself, not just its separate constituents. If new NHS PCTs grasp this nettle then they have the scope and opportunity to respond to the basic human needs of individuals for personal commitment, and as groups to engender a sense of belonging to community (Drucker 1994: pp. 158–161). These needs were once the province of kinship and neighbourhood networks. As local nuclear and extended family relationships diminish, however, policy analysts increasingly recognise the emergent 'virtual' and 'membership' organisations as the principal, if not in some cases the only preferred, option for our tribal identities (Drucker 1994; Hutton 2000; Meads and Ashcroft 2000).

With this option comes the chance to revive the vocational call. The tribe of primary care, given the new breadth of its definition, can have many members and be as diverse and pluralistic as the old professions were narrow and in a standard mould. Such successful enterprises in other sectors, such as Virgin, IBM and even Shelter and Manchester United plc, have already made the necessary changes. In adapting to the wider range of normative as well as calculative needs and expectations that today's men and women bring as employees, contractors and subcontractors, they have increased the range of resources available to them as employers by at least equivalent proportions. PCTs will be the principal resource managers of tomorrow's NHS. This management responsibility means as much procuring resources as it does their deployment. By statute, PCTs are corporate bodies with the standing of a company only required to receive a simple majority of their funds from the NHS (NHSE 1999). For those areas in middle England where blunt socioeconomic indicators reveal little deprivation and low levels of disadvantage, a broad-based approach to the new tribalism will be especially important. Capped staffing budgets, prescribing overspends, high demand helplines and little prospect of either Health Action Zone or NHS Beacon site status suggest that collective self-interest will encourage a catholic approach. The broad church of primary care should be open to all kinds of followers and all kinds of offerings.

At national level, the changes are already happening. The days of exclusive negotiating rights with governments of individual Royal Colleges are clearly coming to an end. The health visitors have retitled their national association to encompass 'community practitioners'. The old fundholders have metamorphosed into the National Association of Primary Care. There is a further National Primary Care Learning Association targeting the teachers and training officers, while both the two national 'Alliance' organisations that have emerged from the experience of locality based commissioning, are explicitly multi-professional in their marketing and recruitment drives.

At local levels the tribal task is tougher and genuinely transformational. Too often, doctors, dentists and even nurses appear to be angry with each other, as well as with society beyond. Too often they feel undervalued and under threat. Too often, at the same time, they also seem to feel over-exposed and overstretched. The early days of NHS PCTs have done little to diminish these dichotomous feelings. Indeed the gradation of different levels of PCGs and PCTs, the very different models and rates of progress in the different parts of the UK, and the inexorable demise of NHS Community Trusts have collectively, in our experience, frequently added to the divisions. There are few role models yet of the new world. Visionaries for PCTs and their complex potential are inevitably far less visible and numerous than those who championed the simpler initiatives of an individual practice-based primary care-led NHS in the 1994–97 period. The value of learning how to transfer the learning about creating the new tribalism required is important for those responsible for PCTs and their development. In addition to the commercial ventures listed above, major modern charities, such as Childline and Action Aid have done it. So too have combinations of housing associations and capital development companies. Even the evangelical movement has created its million-plus-people Alpha tribe through a nationwide programme of meals and messages specifically designed to tap into people's unmet needs for commitment and community. The organisations of primary care must do the same. Without the transferable learning of tribalism the tremendous challenge posed by translating the policy of the new NHS into practice could all too easily turn out to be unsustainable.

Summary

Transferable learning is the central theme of this book. Subsequent chapters seek to address those areas where it is especially important that specific usable lessons are learnt in primary care. Its new NHS trusts have the burden of converting central strategic statements into frontline substance at a time when the NHS has severely limited its own capacity for the kinds of organisational development now required. In learning how to address these shortfalls, in learning actually how to address the questions of *How?* in relation to the logistical and operational requirements of those nationally who normally confine themselves simply to questions of *Why?* and *What for?*, those leading contemporary primary care will need to look elsewhere. In this chapter we have begun to look at the scope and sources of transferable learning. These have been deliberately wide-ranging and, we hope, imaginative. Alternative and applicable transnational service models, modern tribes and, above all, the importance of defining *trust* itself with integrity in an increasingly political primary care environment, are all examples of the stimulation that can be found from breaking down the barriers. In transferable learning there is genuine hope for the future.

References

Denham J (19 February 1999) *Primary Care Trusts* (Ministerial letter to NHS Trust and Health Authority Chairs and Chief Executives, and PCG Chairs).

Drucker P (1994) *Post-Capitalist Society.* Butterworth-Heinemann, Oxford.

Eve R and Mares P (2000) *PCG Development: early perceptions from North Sheffield Primary Care Group.* The Centre for Innovation in Primary Care, Sheffield.

Ford HAJ (1974) *Cases on Trusts.* Sweet and Maxwell, London.

Gardner S (1990) *An Introduction to the Law of Trusts.* Clarendon Press, Oxford.

Giddens A (1998) *The Third Way: the renewal of social democracy.* Polity Press, Cambridge.

Griffiths F and Byrne D (1998) General Practice and the new science emerging from the theories of 'chaos' and 'complexity'. *Br J Gen Pract.* **48**: 1697–99.

Griffiths P (1996) *Presidential address.* Institute of Health Service Managers Annual Conference, Birmingham.

Heath I (1995) *The Mystery of General Practice.* Nuffield Provincial Hospitals Trust, London.

Hutton W (Chair, Commission on the NHS) (2000) *New Life for Health.* Vintage, London.

Klein R (1995) *New Politics of the NHS.* Longman, London.

Meads G (1999) Organisational development in primary care. In: J Sims (ed) *Primary Health Care Sciences.* Whurr, London.

Meads G and Ashcroft J (2000) *Relationships in the NHS: bridging the gap.* Royal Society of Medicine Press, London.

NHS Executive (1999) *Primary Care Trusts: financial framework.* Department of Health, London.

Secretary of State (1997) *The New NHS: modern, dependable.* Department of Health, London.

Starfield B (1992) *Primary Care: concept, evaluation and policy.* Oxford University Press, New York.

Wilkin D, Gillam S and Leese B (eds) (2000) *The National Tracker Survey of Primary Care Groups and Trusts: progress and challenges 1999/2000.* National Primary Care Research and Development Centre, Manchester.

CHAPTER 2

Traumas and turning points

For every example of good practice there are too many examples where change has yet to take place. Managers and clinicians across the NHS must make changes happen.[1]

Disengaging from the NHS

The period of GP fundholding can now seem like a remarkable act of faith on the part of government. Trust was genuinely placed, in both its organisational and ethical senses, in the units furthest removed from the centre, closest to the client coal face; and then the distance and the real freedoms that went with it were actually increased through extended powers of self-regulation and direct purchasing. The aim and result were to release the development energies at the level of the individual practice, or local hospital, because this is where changing behaviour really counted and where commitment, whether through extra fees and/or extra services, could really be generated. Diversity and difference ruled. The political tolerance these required now seems to many in primary care a sign of maturity. The advent of primary care trusts (PCTs) and a centrally written national plan signal a com- plete change in direction and attitude.

Those interviewed during the course of the preparation of this text were unanimous that, despite the promise of additional resources, at practice level the establishment of PCG/Ts had often led to widespread professional disengagement from service and clinical development activities. As a result, organisational development had become, at least temporarily, the sole remaining interest area for those still wanting to participate in the wider life of the NHS, and this interest has been largely confined to the few GPs or nurses on PCG/T boards or the various governance subcommittees. What other development has taken place has been mostly at PCG-only levels and while it has been attractive it has, in many ways, been marginal, affecting neither the practice nor the district level services. In one area we visited, for example, a significant list of minor new local community developments was

---

[1] *NHS Plan* 2000: 9.3

set out by a PCG chief executive, including much improved links with the district council over waste disposal and rural public transport. The local GPs and their fieldwork colleagues received the news politely and commended the changes. Then one spoke for all when he said that none of the changes made any difference either to secondary care, or indeed to the individual practice, where the real changes were needed and where the combined constraints of the SaFF and HImP served to stifle grassroots energies and maintain the status quo. Primary care professionals, he felt, no longer had the means or incentives to engage with the process.

In this climate PCGs have repeatedly been described to us as the 'personal creations' of the chairs and chief executives. In some places this seems to have been all they have been. One interviewee memorably and graphically referred to a local PCG about to be subsumed in a merger as 'a foetus not yet fit to be aborted'. Elsewhere, more generously, these 'personal creations' were regarded as sensitive to, and a reflection of, local circumstances and cultures. Leadership has been both situational and individualistic. Reliance on role and authority structures has been rendered redundant in organisations where staffing levels have rarely reached double figures and, as one PCT chief executive asserted, 'The different component parts do not of themselves add up to a coherent whole'.

The same individual was also acutely aware that his function was to 'facilitate' the process through which a 'cultural melting pot' turned into a new type of healthcare organisation in which adult–adult relationships are the defining characteristic. He and his counterparts, in our interviews, were clear that not only would there be casualties but these were a necessary and worthwhile price of the process. One PCG chief executive described himself as the 'safety valve' for the 'deeply conservative patterns of behaviour' of traditional single-handed practitioners and small practices with their feuds and fees. In moving them to PCT status, he felt it was almost like 'parting them from old friends'. Most PCG managers we met were clear that it is the informal rather than the formal systems they need to influence effectively if PCTs are to be effective organisations.

The bringing together of the managerial culture of health authorities, the independent professional business culture of general practice and its associates, and the local service network culture of community trusts and their nurses into a single organisational framework has sharply exposed all the points of difference. Indeed the traumas have come through the surfacing of not just the different formal features but also the fundamentally divergent sub-cultures. Doctors and social workers have different values and beliefs; nurses and GPs have separate histories and actually alternative professional education approaches. Some of those sitting in the PCG/T boardrooms believe in private ownership. Several do not. With PCTs looking to move further into the territory of combined health and social services, this supplementary

'subcultural melting pot' is only likely to simmer more vigorously as voluntary organisations and the independent social care sector are encompassed
within a primary care organisation's commissioning responsibilities.

The growing scale of PCTs, in both geographic and financial terms, is
commonly regarded as a further cause for disengagement at practitioner
level. The organisations may retain primary care in their name but are felt
to have become too large for this to signify the kinds of personal care with
which this term has been conventionally associated. The PCG/T chief
executives we interviewed supported the impression gained from HMG
workshops during the 1999–2000 period that many fieldworkers, whether
GPs, nurses or therapists, have reverted to what was often referred to as
the 'technician' role. Only one of the ten we interviewed individually
mentioned the Primary Care Investment Plan (PCIP) as a vehicle for much
more than consolidation and minor adjustments to terms and conditions of
practitioners. Far from engaging with the holistic language of health
improvement and integrated care systems, they are simply getting on with
seeing the sick, treating the ill and sustaining the growing number of
stressed people.

Into this last category can be placed many of those who joined PCG
boards within the last 18 months only to find themselves in an unexpec-
tedly short-lived organisation. The logic of progression to PCT status is
proving irresistible in most areas, particularly when firmly supported by the
central political direction and the performance requirements of local health
authorities. The consequence is that many PCGs feel as if they are self-
destructing. To some of their members this is a relief. They can return to
their clinical roles. To others it is a disappointment. They felt they would
genuinely be part of a new type of collaborative enterprise and are taken
aback to find that the hierarchic controls of NHS trust management directly
accountable to the national political administration are to apply just as
much, if not more, in primary care, as they do in secondary settings. They
feel trapped, somewhat deceived, and now probably excluded, with the
places for professionals on the PCT boards strictly limited in number.

To a third group, the stress of being in an organisation predestined to
disappear is almost intolerable. One chief executive of a small PCG being
'taken over' by its larger neighbour seeks career counselling and looks to
her former employer, a big acute hospital, as a future refuge. The elation of
being a PCG pioneer has long since gone. A commissioning manager
deployed by the health authority to work for no fewer than three PCGs,
sees the work he has put into developing effective DHA contracts and contracting mechanisms summarily set aside; and plans to return to his native
Welsh valleys. His counterpart, in a rural PCG, resigns. A former fundholding manager, he resents dismantling the extended practice-level services
his previous GPFH tactical initiatives had helped to create. And so on. The

Table 2.1   New primary care organisations and public health prototypes, November 1998

Type	A 'Defence ASSOCIATION'	B 'Friendly SOCIETY'	C 'Executive AGENCY'	D 'Franchised COMPANY'
Status	Professional network	HA subcommittee	Brokers firm	Mixed status public utility
Accountability (to)	DoH/GMSC(GPC)	HA/LMC	Trusts	National/regional regulators
Purpose	To advocate and represent individual general practice interests for growth and survival	To encourage an inclusive approach to local health issues, based on existing practice arrangements	To constrain secondary care and redirect resources to practices	To control majority healthcare resources of local population
Objectives	• To sustain GMS income • To preserve practice configuration • To defend professional autonomy • To respond effectively to local consultations on health issues	• To support HA as principal purchaser of healthcare • To promote primary care teams with GP leadership • To explore opportunities for interpractice collaboration • To maintain district as NHS performance unit	• To realise critical mass of GPs for general medical practice • To set direction for community health services • To explore scope for improved skills substitution and inter-professional working • To resolve secondary/primary care conflicts via inter-clinician deals and trade-offs	• To operate as a corporate organisation in terms of investment and savings • To address population and individual health issues in balance • To gain community acceptance and active endorsement • To radically revise both GMS and HCHS working practices
Management (by)	Liaison GPs and HA middle manager 'links'	Commissioning (non-GPFH) GPs plus HA purchasing/corporate services managers	Former GPFH leads and business managers – from practices and trusts	Senior Community Trust or HA executives, plus 'new' primary care professional leads on primary healthcare

Health strategy	Operational responses to nationally determined policies and contracts	Derived from DPH annual report and profiles of patient demand, augmented by effective individual representation	Intermediate care-based – avoidable A&Es, continuing care, acute episodes etc. Influenced by SSD community care plans	Based on Patient Enrolment Principle – registered population signed up to organisation's Health Business Priorities – as described in trust prospectus
Public health function	Very limited personnel resources, focused on core roles of communicable diseases, HNA etc.	Operationally aligned with HA commissioning directorate. Closely involved in secondary care and clinical effectiveness issues	Promoting public health issues and alliances at strategic levels with unitary authorities, Chambers of Commerce etc. via shared SLAs	Split between overall performance monitoring and outposted advisory roles, leading multi-professional public health networks including health visitors
Information	Extrapolated from national data sources (e.g. ONS, DoH, MDS etc.)	Locality analyses at parish/ward levels by HA based on NHS morbidity and hospital referral categories	Combined with LAs, and based on district council/municipal boundaries including CHS profiles	Built up from practice level HNAs, and combined with A–C, plus literature/research findings
Internal relations (key)	GMSC, individual patients, traditional NHS managers, RCGP (National)	HA members and chief executive, prescribing adviser, Primary Care Alliance, RCGP (regions), hospital consultants	Community Trust service clinicians and managers, social services budget managers, health economists, accountants, voluntary organisations, Association for Primary Care	New Primary Care Trusts National Group, NICE/CHIMP, NHSE, regional offices/assemblies, media and politicians, commercial sector, major providers
Organisational development (category/prospects)	Mules – very poor	Sheep – depends on bottom line performance	Lambs – to the slaughter – in 'no man's land'	Lions – product champions but few and fragile

Source: Meads *et al.* 1999, p. 36.

reality of the new NHS, for a minority at least, does have its traumas, and the illustrations above, of course, do not even touch upon those in, for example, NHS community trusts and health authority purchasing departments, where the organisations are disappearing altogether.

In previous periods of profound change within the UK healthcare system, there has always been an organisation available to pick up the pieces. The regional health authorities have most frequently fulfilled this function, often serving, for example, as a clearing-house for displaced personnel and a source of bridging finance in times of economic difficulties. For general practices going through partnership splits or cashflow crises arising from delayed fee payments, the Family Practitioner Committee played a similar role. The island of stability and succour in a storm is, however, seemingly no part of the new NHS. No single organisational structure is secure. NHS Direct moves the general practice from the frontline to the second stage of the patient pathway. Community trusts disaggregate and disintegrate. The new regulatory responsibilities of health authorities mean that their rapid reduction in numbers can only be a (relatively short) matter of time. Even the top-level leadership of the Department of Health and NHS Executive merges, leaving the latter with precarious prospects for survival. What is there in this environment that represents a secure investment? All of the chief executives we interviewed described the 'disengagement' of the health authorities and their realignment with the central political administration. For the majority this was a painful experience. They felt abandoned, and left without adequate resources to undertake an agenda that the health authority was still setting. For some, however, this change was recognised as essential. They just wanted the health authority to 'let go', to match its actions to its words.

The divide between expressed policy and its espoused practice is a subject to which our earlier studies have already paid considerable attention (e.g. Meads and Ashcroft 2000: pp. 13–22). Table 2.1 details the four types of primary care organisation identified in a 1998 nationwide study of local partnerships between PCGs and health authorities as they developed the initial HImPs.

This typology defined still possesses a currency in 2000–01. In our experience all PCG/Ts are able to identify themselves with one of the models as being their predominant type. At the same time, however, each PCG/T recognises elements of the first two organisations, the 'Defence Association' and the 'Friendly Society' within their boundaries. Some local force field analyses have indicated there are still plenty of sheep and mules around (Lewin 1951). One of the PCG chief executives we interviewed in the present study described the core of his role as seeking to shift the balance of power between the 'joiners' and 'non-joiners'. On occasions, he had felt he was losing the battle, especially when the politics of future PCT configuration had become apparently all-consuming and a major source of professional alienation as a result. In these circumstances the concept of 'brokerage' is one that those responsible for leading the new primary care organisations have repeatedly drawn upon. In this context transferable learning for one interviewee meant referring back to his past social psychology student days. For him the challenge of offering the future PCT as an attractive prospect and alternative to the disengagement meant thinking in psychometric testing terms, with 'resource investigator' (Belbin 1993) the principal qualification for success as a chief executive in these new 'virtual' organisations.

Disengagement then is a real danger for PCTs. Conceived explicitly as vehicles for 'Working Together' (NHSE 1999) the extent to which they create a change agenda at every level from the individual to the organisational inevitably triggers the universal personal reactions of 'fight/flight' (Argyle 1994). Do we stay or do we go? Do we play the game or tip it over? Can we make what is theirs belong to us? For new PCTs it is a fine balance: too large or a critical mass at last; local agents of central direction or community developments; a new set of stakeholders or a conflict of interests; a direct opportunity for professionals to manage the NHS or the indirect means by which they are placed under political control? It is in the answers to questions such as these, and how they are achieved, that the future viability of NHS PCTs appears to rest.

Re-engaging with the NHS

For better or worse, traumas are often turning points. The suffering involved can clear the way, divorcing the past from the future. The learning experiences of the PCG/T chief executives we interviewed, and of local workshop programmes contemporaneously, suggest that this statement can apply to PCTs. The words are not trite. There are major, substantive grounds for optimism. The new organisations still do represent a set of genuine openings for widespread re-engagement with the new NHS, despite the very real range of risks, overload of central operational instructions and fatigue affecting many participants in yet another systemic change process.

Clinical improvement

The reasons to be encouraged are essentially threefold. First, and perhaps most important, is the PCG/T focus on clinical improvements as their transcendent cause. Two chief executives actually went so far as to say that reaching and maintaining this focus was the 'only' way they had held the new organisation together, preventing either rebellions or outright with-drawals by either individuals or practices over the plethora of organisational development issues they encounter – with future PCT configurations at the top of the list. In the final analysis, as a last resort, clinical efficacy does bind professionals together and PCTs appear the best vehicles the NHS has as yet unearthed for this focus. One PCG chief executive went so far as to tell us that, in her view:

> Clinical benefit is ultimately the only reason for a PCT, without it all the awful tensions over finance – over the health authority not trusting us, about which PCG should lead commissioning – would simply not make it worthwhile. The PCT places everything in a superstructure for better evidence-based care.

She had deliberately spent a lot of time with the relevant documentation and literature – in the form of, for example, National Service Frameworks (NSFs) and Clinical Effectiveness Bulletins – so that she could feel competent and confident in developing the management processes required for multi-professional initiatives on clinical improvement.
   A second chief executive expressed himself more succinctly:

> In this area cost-effectiveness is still anathema to some individual GPs and that is not going to change; at least not for a long time. So 'clinical appropriateness' has become an overarching principle. We're now used to spreading individual initiatives PCG-wide, wherever we can.

Examples included a community-based rehabilitation service, and the roll-out of a local short-life individual practice-based Priority Discharge Team into a PCG-wide 'Avoidable Admissions' task force incorporating three local social services department care managers. For this chief executive, the NSFs were seen as the spinal columns of integrated care programmes in which the multiple contributions of different professionals and agencies are seen as the supporting vertebrae. This was a rare and shining illustration of transferable learning, at a relatively sophisticated level, located between the past development work of a health authority and the emergent primary care organisation operating as the true successor in its leadership of local commissioning. More prosaically another chief executive, in an area of predominantly small, under-developed practices, described 'clinical improvement issues' as the only subject on which the PCG could command sufficient attention to host a local educational event.

Relationships management

The second reason for encouragement is that good management is being recognised as an intrinsic component of clinical improvement. What has been described as the skills of really managing healthcare are being rediscovered (Iles 1997). The essence of these skills is the facilitation of right relationships with what Iles termed the 'generosity' and 'discipline' they require (pp. 78–88). This style of management is a service. It is characterised by a strength of conviction on the one hand, and a sense of humility on the other. It recognises that enduring improvements are much more likely if they are rooted in value-based behaviours than transitional organisational structures and their transitory occupational roles. Relationships management of the prospective PCT is far-removed from the not-so-distant NHS epochs of general management and market regulation. Those we have worked with who were appointed to PCT roles with senior responsibilities during these last periods have often found the adjustments required of them by contemporary primary care organisations hard to make. Some are clearly unsuited in temperament to make them. Others, of course, welcome the changes. They are able to reveal a different side of themselves and are more at ease gaining their legitimacy in an NHS where authority is earned locally rather than conferred from above.

One chief executive expressed this feeling with a degree of lyricism:

> My primary care group is a hollow organisation. It only exists, and performs as a function of the relationships and networks it has. It has become the voice box for a strategy that is owned by the local providers, social services, the district council and the local players. We just pull it together. They use us as the honest broker. We deliver it on their behalf. My role is to make sure we are the expression of our constituents, of each and all of the stakeholders.

His counterparts elsewhere expressed similar sentiments. One stressed the relative importance of interpersonal skills vis-à-vis his formal role. Another saw the PCG's absolute commitment to its local community as the source of a single community approach actually within the PCG itself as it moves to trust status over the next nine months. In this context the chief executive saw the pattern of relationships between the PCT staff, supporters and sub-contractors constituting a single mutually reinforcing pattern of interdependent relationships. It was this kind of pattern that a third chief executive had in mind when she commented on the potential strengths, and shortfalls, of future relationship-based PCTs:

A PCG/T is genuinely a healthcare organisation not an illness institution. We haven't had these in the NHS before and it is hard for those who have worked in it a long time to get to grips with the difference. In my time at this PCG I have seen the full extremes of functionality and dysfunctionality as a result.

The recognition of the value and practical significance of relationships has already proved an important source for both conscious and unconscious learning. In one PCG area a pattern of leadership pairings on all key development issues had been established with the chair and chief executive modelling the behaviour of an effective duo through their visibly close work together, their joint presentations, and their united messages. The pairings were adroitly and informally engineered to take forward, for example, clinical governance, an IM&T strategy and integrated care management. The pairings included an opinion-leading GP and his community nurse counterpart, a representative of fundholding and a friendly non-fundholding GP, and a community health authority accountant with a more sceptical doctor on the SaFF consultation. The pattern was crystal clear, but was actually almost a surprise to the chief executive when revealed. His transferable learning was from a previous role at the political interfaces of NHS performance management and at best semi-conscious. His response to seeing the reflection of his own style was to describe 'relationships management' as 'a way of thinking'.

What one chief executive described as 'a really good ear for those rumours you need to put straight straightaway' and personal intuition, whatever its origins, are, however, not enough, and PCG/Ts have turned to a range of relationship managing techniques for assistance. Some of the more robust of these are described in Chapters 4 and 6; and Table 2.2 provides a worked example based on an early 2000 workshop of how one PCG found the use of popular sports team models useful in both addressing its functions and achieving a modicum of corporacy. For this organisation in transition it was vital to find a framework which allowed corporacy to develop on a basis other than complete unanimity or full participation in the process. Primary care professionals historically have not been accustomed to taking collective action, particularly at local level. This method is based originally on action research with SSD teams 20 years ago, in the days when neighbourhood social work was the radical innovation (Payne 1982). It remains simple and effective today. The relational issues are much the same; the learning from one context across two decades to parallel circumstances is, therefore, deceptively straightforward as a result.

On the whole an explicit willingness to employ theory into practice perspectives has been rare among the PCG/T senior managers and professionals we have encountered. References to constant 'fire fighting', 'operational pressures' and 'feeding the beast' have meant most have been unable in one interviewee's words 'to peel back more than a single layer of the onion ring'. This closed outlook is one reason why several have felt over-whelmed; imprisoned by the day, and captured by the centralising machinery of government. One glorious exception was a PCG chief executive who felt completely on terms with his role and quoted organisational development principles almost as a mantra:

> Form follows function.
>
> Purpose, vision and values first (and this is vital in a clinically-led organisation).
>
> Structure and process must run together. In PCG/Ts they must shape one another. Never think of them in linear terms, as a sequence.

Here was an individual who had always seen 'organisational health' as a chief executive's first and peculiar responsibility, whatever the setting. For him the advent of PCG/Ts was a long-awaited opportunity to put the thoughts of Beckhard and Harris (1987), Berwick (1991), and their like on organisational change and quality into practice, through working together on the positive relationships required 'to convert individual inventors into collective innovators'. As a result the PCG's lowest common denominator had moved up a notch from specific clinical improvements to generalisable service developments. Its role was defined not as a fixed organisation in its own right but as a dynamic component of what was termed 'the local health economy'. The PCG chief executive actually defined himself not as a prospective NHS trust general manager but as one of those 'offering leadership to and in a healthcare system'. Interestingly, this same chief executive only planned to stay with the PCG/T for a short while. Part of his clarity about his 'change agent' role came from his certainty about his future. He would give it a couple of years, deliver the PCT, and move on. For all his sophistication in terms of organisational development, he felt the New NHS was 'a hell of a change, a hell of a challenge, going at a hell of a pace'. And he would shortly have had enough.

Local alliances

The new primary care organisations often find themselves being more popular outside the NHS than within it. For many they represent a threat to the long-established order and, certainly, it is not unusual for prospective PCTs to place local authorities before health authorities in their lists of

Table 2.2 Corporate team metaphors (examples)

Type	Characteristics	PCT applications
Cricket	Aggregate of individual specialists (e.g. opening batsman, fast bowler, first slip); complementary skills	Board ownership of individual initiatives (e.g. on IT, alternative therapies) by whole, inclusion of mavericks, 'a place for everyone'
Tennis	In pairs, usually mixed doubles, with changing personnel	Creation of 'club' culture, combinations on interface issues (e.g. clinical governance, communications, care management) between nurse/ GP, SSD/lay representatives etc.
Football	Three-tiers: defence, midfield and attack; one ball; most goals in the net wins, strong co-ordinating coach vital	GP chair and aggressive personality types are released to be strikers; no own-goals by a solid back four (clinical governance, financial control, prescribing, waiting lists); executive officers operate in midfield fetching and carrying, making the passes
Rugby	Separate forwards and backs, linked by scrum-half, hooker and props vital in obtaining ball, touch down tries over the line	Placing big 'hitters' in right positions; using innovative practices as flying wings and finance managers as hookers to win resources, linking solidity on internal functions and performance monitoring with flexibility and mobility on service development
Basketball	High-scoring, integrated team, attacking and defending as one unit with constant set positions and plays, substitutes slip seamlessly on to court	Model for transition to real PCT working as a corporate entity; with agreed skills mix, single employer arrangements, vocal supporters and ready substitutions

prospective partners. Across the country, in the sites we have visited during the 1998–2000 period, local authorities and their social services departments have generally embraced PCG/Ts as a new opportunity for collaboration. Politically led, especially in areas where the unitary version applies, local authority officers have exercised a basic political judgement about the New NHS and what it means for them. The judgement is that real power is shifting in two directions: first towards a broader role for public health; and secondly in favour of the resource base for secondary care. This is how they read such signals as the reorganisation of the Department of Health with, for example, a single chief officer for the NHS and Social Services, a second deputy chief medical officer now heading the Health Services Directorate, and the NHS Plan's announcement of 7000 extra beds, 7500 more consultants (compared with only 2000 more GPs), 20 000 extra nurses and, of course, 100 new hospitals. To be in on the action means being part of the commissioning function for this growing resource base. It means ensuring the language of 'health inequalities' gets translated into special needs social care programmes. Ultimately, for local authorities and for many local non-statutory organisations as well, it means redefining themselves.

In three of the PCG areas we worked with in preparing this book, SSDs began to rename their staff with the generic title 'primary care workers'. Local alliances with PCG/Ts are not just about altruism. Collaboration, co-ordination and co-operation are fine words. It has been encouraging to witness the principles of partnership apply in straightforward practical ways in terms of, for example, improved child protection procedures or elderly at-risk registers. In the words of one PCG chief executive we interviewed, this has amounted to basic common sense: 'Without the alliances we don't mean anything – because we don't deliver anything of ourselves'.

The bottom lines, however, are self-interest and self-preservation. NHS PCTs are seen by their new local allies as the only option, politically, for sustaining a robust, coherent community services infrastructure in relation to a much-strengthened medically-oriented secondary care sector. To be robust and coherent this community services infrastructure must be integrated across its provider roles. It can no longer afford its separate professional aspirations and identities. It must speak with one voice. PCTs must really utilise their position at the frontline and exploit the power of this unique perspective in being able to serve as the mechanism for controlling supply and demand. This means, of course, no longer simply relying on the separate general practices as gatekeepers but incorporating these with all the other referral points into a viable resource and demand management system. The *NHS Plan* recognises the need for this fundamental change itself. It is NHS Direct not the general medical practitioner, for example, which is now described as 'a one-stop gateway to healthcare' (1.11); and the proposed new Care Trusts have as their *raison d'être* the 'even closer integration of health and social services'. The purpose of their 'broader role' is:

> To establish new single multi-purpose legal bodies to commission and be responsible for all local health and social care. (Secretary of State 2000: 7.9)

That such a change can be proposed now with a degree of real confidence is a tribute to the ways in which many of those responsible for leading the new primary care organisations have exercised their leadership roles. They have put aside the conventional NHS organisational doctrines of hierarchy, bureaucracy, separate professions and even general management. Networks, mentors, directors without portfolio and, above all, virtual organisations occupy their new mental maps. One chief executive we interviewed explicitly drew on human geography principles. On several other occasions the names of Virgin, Microsoft and even Burger King were cited as virtual organisational models to emulate in their use of franchising arrangements, small semi-autonomous subsidiaries, clear overall strategic objectives and quality management techniques. In the past the integration of health and social services was the poisoned chalice, passed swiftly on to joint planning officers in health and local authorities located on the margins of their organisations. Now the boundary players have been moved centre stage. A well-managed PCG/T is a complex system of local alliances with flexible project managers sustaining their development dynamic through the constant input of new ideas and interests, and a sustained output of disseminated learning and cross-sectoral service programmes. Nominally these project managers may have a variety of employers: the community trust, an SSD, the health authority or even the likes of Age Concern or Help the Aged. In the past, as one PCT chief executive politely put it:

> These different parts have had their distinctive characteristics, which at all costs they have wanted to hold onto. As a virtual organisation our job in a PCT requires facilitative management. We can make sure now they all add up to a single whole. The press is watching what we do (on NHS and local authority issues) and we can really use this counter-media thrust to keep all the troops on board.

In short, in private and in public, PCTs are the opportunity for a fresh start, and the scale of their early local alliances is the best evi- dence of this new beginning.

A virtual organisation as a theoretical construct does have its own defining characteristics. These include a small number of simple overarching aims with which there are high levels of internal and external identification; a strong commitment from personnel beyond that of their host employer; substantial subsidiarity in roles and responsibilities for operational resource management; and the use of unifying standardised quality systems. While, however, the term 'virtual organisation' was frequently used by our interviewees, it was not often employed with this degree of definitional clarity. Rather, it was employed in a general sense, as if referring to a movement paving the way for the organisation yet to come. In this sense future Care Trusts will be the fulfilment of a mission. For the time being, however, Figure 2.1 captures the usual image of PCG/Ts as virtual organisations. It comes from the same chief executive who identified organisational health as his role's first and peculiar responsibility.

As Figure 2.1 indicates, the PCT can open doors and is itself emerging as an open door for participation. Providing much more space to come together, both formally and informally, enhances not simply operational contacts but strategic processes as well. PCTs create the forums for what are described in Chapter 4 as authentically 'emergent' strategies; i.e. the discernible results and patterns of combined behaviour over time. This form of strategy is much stronger than its predecessors. It has a deeper and wider ownership than rational planning. Its value base is altogether more robust and outcome oriented than strategies derived solely from market mechanisms. It is far less politicised than those strategic statements made for positional and publicity purposes.

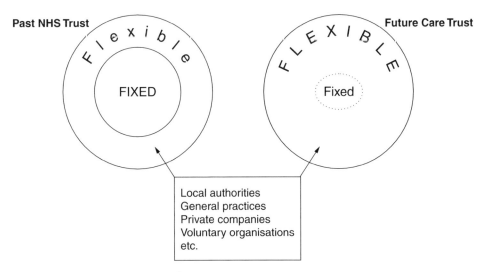

Figure 2.1   Becoming a virtual organisation.

Box 2.1 is an illustration of the stages of management in the kinds of strategic process now available to PCTs. This 'network-based' model is derived from a parallel local study of local primary eye care develop-ments in a central London area. It indicates how the leadership of primary care organisations have the chance to generate new and valued contributions to locally instigated strategic initiatives from across the health and social care system with, for example, consultants as educators, social workers as care co-ordinators, managers as facilitators and peer professionals as regulators.

Box 2.1   Primary care: network-based development

1 Market development – business collaboration on training, informa-tion and marketing to expand overall service sector.
2 Joint training – based on common ground of maintaining clinical standards and maximising individuals' skills.
3 Specialist accreditation – to legitimise development, and enlist support of key secondary care and academic 'leads'.
4 Shared monitoring and review – expanding peer mechanisms for professionals with management oversight to ensure overall com-pliance with health policies.
5 Joint facilitation – by partnership between individual professional and executive representatives personally modelling approach to strategic change and acting as catalyst throughout service development.

Source: Meads 1999, p. 275

The virtual organisation model is an ideal vehicle for local alliances. It gives permission to become a stakeholder in the future, and releases prisoners from the past. These local alliances, sustained by an effective relationships management approach, and balanced by a bottom line practice concern for clinical improvements are proving the main determinants of PCTs' development in their early stages. These are not insignificant gains for primary care over what went before. The rhetoric, however, for PCTs is still often about rather more. It proclaims PCTs as champions of community health and development, as conduits of evidence-based medicine and healthcare, as expressions of interprofessional learning, and as the main means of restoring public confidence in a revitalised NHS. New primary care organisations at the beginning of 2001 are a long way from being all these things. Their 'modernisation' agenda remains immense. For them to match the central rhetoric to local realities through their new resource management responsibilities is a huge challenge. It is to this dimension of the relationship between policy and practice that we must now turn our attention to complete our scene-setting role in the first section of this handbook.

References

Argyle M (1994) *The Psychology of Interpersonal Behaviour* (5e). Penguin, London.

Beckhard R and Harris R (1987) *Organisational Transitions: managing complex change* (2e). Addison Wesley, London.

Belbin M (1993) *Team Roles at Work.* Butterworth-Heinemann, Oxford.

Berwick D (1991) *Curing Health Care: new strategies for quality improvement.* Jossey Bass, San Francisco.

Iles V (1997) *Really Managing Healthcare.* Open University Press, Buckingham.

Lewin K (1951) *Field Theory in Social Sciences.* Harper and Row, New York.

Meads G (1999) Streaming into the river. *J Interprofessional Care.* **13**: 3.

Meads G, Killoran A, Ashcroft J and Cornish Y (1999) *Mixing Oil and Water.* HEA Publications, London.

Meads G and Ashcroft J (2000) *Relationships in the NHS: bridging the gap.* Royal Society of Medicine Press, London.

NHS Executive (1999) *Working Together: human resources guidance and requirements for primary care trusts.* Department of Health, London.

Payne M (1982) *Working in Teams.* Macmillan, Basingstoke.

Secretary of State (2000) *NHS Plan.* Department of Health, London.

CHAPTER 3

Rhetoric, resources and realities

Now, the necessary resources are in place.[1]

The insider perspective

The preceding chapters have offered in turn horizontal and vertical perspectives on PCTs as the new organisational means for translating central policy into local practice. The lateral viewpoints from other non-NHS organisations and different healthcare systems in Chapter 1 have been followed by the juxtaposition between the expression of formal policy statements and the experience of actual fieldwork in Chapter 2. This chapter offers a third, internal perspective, pragmatically assessing the resource management options of PCTs as they assume their new mandates. Both the scope and the constraints represented by this perspective are recurring themes in the subsequent chapters of this book. New resources of themselves do not, for example, offer automatic answers to the divergence of public health and primary care described in Chapter 5, or to the removal of the 'antagonistic' and 'handmaiden' models of PCG/SSD relationships analysed in Chapter 6. These stem from deep-rooted attitudinal differences and divergent cultures, with their origins in educational selection. In such circumstances, more resources can simply consolidate a condition. More resources can mean more problems. That PCTs can respond to political rhetoric through realistic resource management strategies and tactics is an essential prerequisite of their change agent role. Adopting an inside-out perspective on what is possible for them to achieve in terms of the efficient use of resources constitutes the basic litmus test for not only their viability but for many of the New NHS policy proposals and plans.

From our work with PCG/Ts over the past two years this insider perspective produces four such tests. The first two have an intra-organisational

---

[1] *NHS Plan* 2000: 16.11

bias for a PCT. The second pair respond to the new trusts' external expectations and requirements. In summary they are:

- *Probity*. The PCT must be secure and safe on its statutory, financial and clinical responsibilities, particularly in the context of new governance requirements and multiple stakeholder accountabilities. This probity must be systematic and demonstrable, preferably through visible successes on issues of dishonesty and malpractice.
- *Information systems*. The PCT must be in a position to meet its account-abilities and hold its constituents to account, through the regular, consistent supply of relevant information from and between each of its participant levels: practitioner, practice, inter-practice co-operative ven-tures, locality partnership agencies and PCT/inter-PCT functions.
- *Resource utilisation*. The PCT is responsible for ensuring effective and efficient management of resources both in its territory and for its territory within the wider health and social care systems. On the use of therapeutics and other providers, in particular, it must be able to undertake the appropriate analyses and assessments, with the means of promoting better value through alternative incentives across its associated family health, social and acute service providers.
- *Performance management*. The PCT is nationally the new pivotal unit of NHS performance. A basic stipulation is to meet all the monitoring require-ments of either NHS approved independent regulatory or supervisory bodies and to maximise the level of PCT 'modernisation' resources for development as a result.

This chapter will examine each of the above in turn, drawing on specific examples from our research as illustrations and examples of good practice, where relevant. This specific insider perspective is a hard-headed one: what can work and will it?

Probity

PCTs operate within a prescribed framework of corporate governance and probity (NHS Executive 1999a). The PCT Board, which consists of a lay chair and a majority of non-executives, is responsible for providing strate-gic oversight and verification to the day-to-day management role of the Executive Committee, where professional members will be in the majority. The Board must ensure that the key requirements of public accountability, probity and public involvement are fully met.

Investments need to be made in accordance with the requirements laid down in Standing Orders and Standing Financial Institutions and the decision-making process needs to be open, to prevent conflicts of interest and take account of public opinion. PCTs must adhere to the formal codes of conduct, accountability and openness. This is particularly important, for example, in respect of GMS and local development scheme reimbursements where the income of individual practices is affected. Appropriate consultations also need to be made with the Local Medical Committee (LMC) in accordance with statutory and informal good practice requirements.

PCTs should ensure that minimum control standards are in place with satisfactory budgetary disciplines, safeguarding of assets and an internal audit function. These provide for the controlling and monitoring of expenditure and assets, and protect individuals through adequate and clear lines of delegated responsibility.

The above framework mirrors that of health authorities which in turn have strengthened their governance arrangements following the publication of the Cadbury Report in 1992 (Cadbury 1992). The PCT Board needs access to robust and timely information to ensure that it can fulfil its duties of public accountability and probity. Risks need to be identified openly: whether relating to clinical, financial, performance monitoring or organisational issues. As a result they can then be avoided, if possible, or detected and dealt with if they occur.

PCTs are also significant players in the drive against fraud and corruption within the NHS. The remit of the Directorate of Counter Fraud Services (DCFS) within the NHS Executive is:

> To have overall responsibility for all work to counter fraud and corruption within the NHS with particular priority for countering fraud in the Family Health Services. (Department of Health 1998/231)

The aim is to reduce fraud to an absolute minimum within ten years This means putting in place arrangements to hold fraud at a minimum level permanently, to enable more NHS resources to be directed at providing better patient care.

One of the first targets of the DCFS has been to identify and reduce loss in the family health services. Prescription fraud by both patients and contractors is a key issue. The introduction of point of dispensing checks by pharmacy contractors from 1 April 1999 is estimated to have resulted in a reduction in losses from patient charge evasion of £36 million (Department of Health press release, 17 March 2000). PCTs need to be aware of ongoing developments in this area. Repeat prescribing systems may be a source of weakness in individual practices and open to abuse by dishonest contractors, particularly in respect of nursing and residential home prescribing where audit trails are often poor. Losses in this area can have a major impact on prescribing expenditure and PCT prescribing advisers need to review Prescribing Analysis and Cost (PACT) data provided through the Prescription Pricing Authority (PPA) for any adverse trends which may be due to fraud.

PCTs face a complex and difficult task in ensuring that the requirements of corporate governance and probity are met. Interests need to be declared, and donations recorded. Decisions must be open and justifiable. With multiple stakeholders, this is a demanding agenda but one of critical importance if PCTs are to be publicly accountable bodies. This accountability in the New NHS is much more complicated than before. In practical financial terms 'stakeholding' means different sources of investment, each requiring robust but distinct reporting arrangements. Local authority grants, corporate sponsorship, individual dowries, NHS revenue, private capital and so on: the importance of having explicit arrangements for probity, given this potential for 'mess' and 'messing up', can scarcely be overstated. The preliminary financial framework guidance for PCTs, not surprisingly, ran to as many as 34 pages, spawning six further supporting documents in the next 12 months (NHSE 1999b).

Information systems

PCT Accountability Agreements with health authorities contain performance targets ranging from childhood immunisation rates, to in-patient and day-case waiting lists, to average generic prescribing rates per GP. Understanding the key variables which lie beneath the achievement of these targets which, in turn, underpin the six areas of the National Plan, will be a crucial task for PCTs. The six areas identified personally by the Prime Minister are:

- patient access
- patient empowerment
- partnership
- professions/workforce
- performance
- prevention.

(*NHS Plan*: Preface, p. 1)

The fulfilment of the PCT task is dependent on their access to, and interpretation of, the information sources available.

For PCTs, with their unique capacity to see healthcare systems as a whole, from the individual to the population perspective, information really is power. PCTs need to understand the link between the referral patterns, prescribing and clinical protocols of their constituent practices, and such measured targets as outpatient or in-patient waiting lists for treatment and emergency admissions.

There are many factors to be taken into account. Health Service Circular 1999/065 provides guidance on the implementation of clinical governance (Department of Health 1999/065). It emphasises that the routine availability of sound information for monitoring and benchmarking purposes is essential if the quality of care is to be improved. There is a need for systematic work within PCTs to assess and enhance the quality and completeness of data held in clinical systems in order to make informed use of the aggregate information, to support both clinical governance and audit and commissioning decisions.

Clinical systems are now urgently needed to develop and support the user needs of all primary healthcare team (PHCT) members − GPs, practice nurses, therapists and other community workers − so that data has to be entered only once and then shared with authorised users to provide such details as symptoms, diagnoses, treatments, test results, medication, care plans and expected and actual outcomes. Here the transferable learning from the IT-based systems of developing countries, such as those described in Chapter 1, is obvious.

PCTs have a responsibility to focus on evidence-based clinical practice, to support and incentivise good practice, and to improve clinical standards at local levels. To meet these responsibilities they need to engage in comparative performance monitoring between practices, to look at outliers and discuss and apply peer professional pressure as an expression of the new managerialism now expected of previously autonomous clinicians, where appropriate (Harrison 1999).

PCTs have the ability, through the investment of both GMS and Modernisation Fund IT resources, to develop common information databases. They are able to do this through the use of communication links and data exchange between practice-based and PHCT IT systems and to provide the required integration. They are now, for the first time, in a position to develop the means to access, aggregate, analyse and act on data to support the planning, commissioning, monitoring and evaluation of health and healthcare services from a meaningful primary care site. Each of these elements of a comprehensive IM&T infrastructure, according to central guidance, should be covered from March 2001 in a PCT's Local Implementation Strategy (LIS) (NHSE 2000).

PCTs require access to detailed information on the care provided to their patients by NHS trusts and other organisations. This includes reports on: both emergency and elective admissions; finished consultant episodes where the registered practice of the patient is identified; length of stay distributions by specialty, levels of activity compared with those planned in service agreements, and comparable time periods in previous years. PCTs need information on outpatient care, the use of Accident and Emergency services by their patients and the regular validation of patients on waiting lists. This information is critical to their new role as custodians for efficient resource utilisation in their whole health economies.

PCTs should look at practice-level data to create practice profiles, using practice demographics to 'normalise' data, and to compare analytically with both the impact on secondary care and to the aggregate targets achieved. They must constantly seek to understand cause and effect and they are especially well placed to do this. Primary care data relating to the local incidence of diseases and conditions, and inequalities in access should also increasingly inform and determine the contents of the Health Improvement Plan (HImP).

In looking at primary care data there are other factors to be taken into account, including the impact of local development schemes within individual practices or on a patch basis, investment in practice staff, the development of such services as practice-based physiotherapy and counsellors, links with the voluntary sector and collaboration with local authority initiatives. All of these contribute to the bigger picture of what options are available for individual patients in response to their needs. PCTs really do have a fresh scope to address the wastelands of duplication and divergence, from practice to district levels.

Detailed prescribing data is available through PACT information supplied by the PPA. Prescribing advisers can evaluate and monitor prescribing in their area by sorting and summation at different organisational levels, time periods and formulary categories. In addition, information is available on potential generic savings, high cost drugs initiated in secondary care, and on comparisons with other PCTs with similar socio-demographic population profiles.

In harnessing this information, in trying to piece the jigsaw together and in seeking to understand the impact on patient wellbeing and the demands on secondary care provision, PCTs have a resource of paramount importance. It is fundamental to their tasks of making informed investment and disinvestment decisions, and supporting clinical governance requirements. PCT investment inevitably will be in the best practice(s); it will not necessarily represent equality of investment. The use of this information by PCTs for efficiency at levels beyond the practice will clearly change the basic parameters in England of primary care itself.

Resource utilisation

PCTs will have substantial resources at their disposal which have to be made to work in the most productive ways if PCTs are to maximise their potential in improving health and healthcare for the local population. The scale of the resources by themselves, however, is deceptive. They are subject to constraints in their use far removed from GP fundholding (GPFH) style commercial freedoms and driving best value for each pound within real public regulatory constraints is a challenge for PCT leaderships.

As Chapter 8 illustrates, PCTs have a unified resource budget covering Hospital and Community Health Services (HCHS), prescribing and General Medical Services (GMS) expenditure to purchase and provide (at level 4) services on behalf of their managed populations.

Unified budgets have been set to reflect previous baseline activity and by reference to weighted capitation target shares which, in turn, have been determined through a national formula designed to allocate resources according to the health needs of the population. The main bulk of resources inherited by PCTs will, therefore, be fed into historic spending patterns in relation to service agreements for hospital services, prescribing expenditure and individual practice reimbursements for staff and IT support.

HCHS monies are committed through the Service and Financial Framework (SaFF) process. In this PCTs are participants alongside local NHS trusts and the health authority in assessing the competing demands of service developments, cost pressures, efficiency gains, etc. Even resources committed to NHS trusts outside the local SaFF process will be aggregated and distributed centrally as part of the distribution of out-of-area treatment (OAT) resources to other host authorities. PCTs may endeavour to cut OAT referrals but the majority (80%) reflect emergency admissions over which the PCT actually has almost no control.

Initial flexibilities for PCTs will, therefore, be very much at the margins of HCHS expenditure with investments directed at locally tailored services either within NHS trusts, or with private providers, or in the development of primary care facilities. PCTs and their frontline clinicians will be key players in negating the assumption that new clinical developments automatically lead to increased or enhanced secondary care provision. For example, one first wave PCT we encountered has used HCHS resources at the margins to occupy an under-used facility and develop a local pain relief service for patients with muscular/skeletal difficulties, offering consultant and physiotherapy input as well as the use of complementary medicines. The aim is to provide a possible alternative to conventional drug regimes and for a small team to consider the individualised needs of referred patients. This is a forerunner to the development of locality care centres within the geographic area offering out-patient clinics, diagnostic facilities and treatments for minor injuries which will require, over time, a much more substantial planned input of resources from growth or redeployment.

Both the accumulated and underlying deficits of many acute NHS trusts will mitigate against the redeployment of resources to locality and primary care developments. In the early years of PCTs the main changes may, as a result, have to come through dialogue between clinicians about how the bulk of the HCHS resources committed by the PCT through the SaFF process are used in local trusts, given the strategic directions agreed within the HImP. PCTs need to be able to really 'own' their referrals and see their costs fairly reflected in the value of their service agreements. Block service agreements provide stability within the health economy and minimise in-year financial risk to PCTs, but they also minimise flexibility unless there is also a significant responsiveness in-year to allow 'unspent' resources to be recycled to meet other priorities, which can be provided at marginal or variable cost.

PCTs can also utilise growth to develop services within practices to impact on the need for secondary care provision in the extension of GMS provision through local development schemes. The latter also address inequalities in service provision, as in Central Southampton PCG's quality award-winning coronary health disease programme operated by constituent practices. This scheme sought to meet diverse cultural needs, and was achieved through partnerships involving patients, carers, the local trust and health authority. It was actually project-managed by a pharmaceutical company. In addition, the project also led to a service agreement between the PCG and two clinical directorates at the local trust which specified outcomes for both secondary and primary care provision. These focused on the patient's perspective of NHS care as one continuum.

HCHS resources may also be used in the primary care setting to provide clinical assistant sessions to tackle particular waiting list priorities. This has been used, for example, to particular effect in a number of locations where HMG associates have worked in respect of dermatology, ophthalmology and audiology. In each case substitution is leading to a better skill mix and a better return on the PCT's investment.

Section 31 of the Health Act 1999 allows the NHS and local authorities (covering all health-related functions, i.e. education, leisure, environment, housing and transport, as well as social services), to delegate commissioning and providing functions to the voluntary sector where this will improve the quality of services. Within PCTs, resources specifically ear-marked for Health Improvement Partnership Grants and voluntary organisations will be small but use can be made of them to support HImP objectives, particularly those relevant to the locality. The sharing of protocols of care and a common language and understanding will be crucial if significant resources are to be pooled to advance local healthcare delivery. Special placements, for example, are a significant financial risk to PCTs and are one area where increased co-operation between agencies, and the increased flexibilities afforded by the 1999 Act, may enable a redirection of energies to allow both a more satisfactory outcome for individual patients and better value for money for their commissioning agents.

The unit of the PCT can provide a focal point to initiate such developments. It is critically dependent on the drive of individuals seeking a better deal for their patients to break down the barriers that the degrees of flexibility within the unified budget allows. The recognition of need, user-clinical dialogue and clinical drive, knowledge and understanding are the key components in offsetting the constraints imposed by the management of the whole health economy, as reflected in the SaFF process and in associated centralised planning. These sources of support will, of course, become still more powerful if the PCT can demonstrate the kind of public legitimacy described in Chapters 4 and 15 and use its 'company' and 'community organisation' status to gain a range of financial sponsors from the community to augment its national taxation-based funding.

Performance management

PCTs are one of the new pivotal units of NHS performance. The NHS Performance Assessment Framework published in June 1999 (NHSE 1999c) introduced a broader-based approach to assessing performance in the NHS. 'Performance is no longer judged just by the numbers of patients treated or the efficiency of services but also by the quality of services provided to deliver the best results for patients and their families.' (CIPFA 1999: Section 5). In this, six dimensions of the healthcare system were identified:

• health improvement
• fair access
• efficiency
• effective delivery of appropriate healthcare
• patient/carer experience
• health outcomes.

Accountability agreements are the basis on which PCTs are performance managed by their host health authorities. They, in turn, are performance managed by their respective NHSE regional office. Key performance targets ranging from numbers of patients and admissions to numbers of referrals, immunisation coverage and generic prescribing rates are reflected at each level.

Meeting performance targets should be seen as a desirable aim for PCTs as a vehicle for utilising local resources and information to best effect, and making primary and secondary care facilities really work for the benefit of patients and their families. In this sense each central target is a local development opportunity.

PCTs and their partners in the health economy have the opportunity through dialogue, negotiation and agreement to influence and change the pattern of service provision where it would be advantageous to do so. The flexibilities afforded by the unified budget, pooled budgets with local authorities, the provision of services by voluntary organisations, and local development schemes, need to be used imaginatively if performance targets are to be attained. In seeking to understand the complex relationship between cause and effect in the healthcare system, PCTs will be better equipped to direct or redirect resources to maximum benefit than any of their NHS predecessors.

Bridging the gap

As an example, locality care centres may impact on outpatient waiting lists; community care provisions by the PCTs and collaborative arrangements with social services may reduce delayed discharges for people aged 75 or over, which in turn will impact on in-patient/day-case waiting lists. The opportunities are there. Appropriate funding is vital but funding is not the only resource which can be made to work to achieve targets: clinical practice, organisational arrangements and the utilisation of existing facilities all need to be considered. PCTs are uniquely well placed to be the fulcrum around which the different forces of the local health and social care system can be rebalanced to achieve the right direction of travel.

The chapters that follow in Part 2 examine just how specific services opportunities may be accepted. They demonstrate how the robust approach to resource management outlined in this chapter needs to be matched throughout a PCT's full range of responsibilities if the transferable learning on offer is to successfully convert rhetoric into realities. They can help to bridge the gap.

References

Cadbury (Committee chair) (1992) *Report on the Financial Aspects of Corporate Governance.* Gee and Co., London.

Chartered Institute of Public Finance and Accountancy (1999) *Financial Information Service, Volume 30.* CIPFA, London.

Harrison S (1999) Clinical autonomy and health policy: past and futures. In: M Exworthy and F Halford (eds) *Professionals and the New Managerialism.* Open University Press, Buckingham, pp. 50–64.

Health Service Circular (1998/231) *Countering Fraud in the NHS*. Department of Health, London.

Health Service Circular (1999/065) *Clinical Governance in the New NHS*. Department of Health, Wetherby.

NHS Executive (1999a) *Primary Care Trusts: establishment, the preparatory period and their functions*. Department of Health, London.

NHS Executive (1999b) *Primary Care Trust: financial framework*. Department of Health, Leeds.

NHS Executive (1999c) *The NHS Performance Assessment Framework*. Department of Health, Wetherby.

NHS Executive (2000) *IM&T Requirements to Support Primary Care Groups and Primary Care Trusts*. Department of Health, Leeds.

PART 2

Practice into policy

Health Management Group and Associates

CHAPTER 4

Releasing the dividend of 'new' partnerships

John Ashcroft

> *Ideological boundaries or institutional barriers should not be allowed to stand in the way of better care.*[1]

The emergence of primary care groups (PCGs) and subsequently primary care trusts (PCTs) has seen significant changes in the number and nature of their relationships, both within these new primary care organisations as well as in their external relationships. This chapter draws on the lessons of working with over 50 PCGs to explore the issues facing PCTs as they seek to release the dividends of new partnerships.[2]

'New' partnerships – the changing relational map

A new context

The New NHS White Paper (Secretary of State for Health 1997) established a 'duty of partnership' between organisations and professions in the provision of healthcare. The concern for partnership is, however, neither new nor restricted to healthcare. Collaboration between health and social services, for example, is a concern as old as the NHS with varying forms and degrees of partnership working being developed over the years. Public services have been giving, for example, increased attention to partnerships with contractors and suppliers as part of 'best value' contracting. Public private partnerships (PPPs) are a major source of investment in public services.

---

[1] *NHS Plan,* 2000: 11.2
[2] This chapter draws on material from the Relational Health Care Project – many of whose projects have been a partnership between the Relationships Foundation and City University's Health Management Group. This work is written up more fully in Meads and Ashcroft 2000.

Partnering has been actively promoted by the Department of Trade and Industry (DTI) in the construction industry to reduce both construction time and costs.

New boundaries

Partnerships are part of the concern for the modernisation of public services, characterised by joined-up government and integrated and accessible services. Increasingly the independence and separateness of the parties to partnership is no longer an unquestioned starting point. There is the prospect of potentially far-reaching changes to both the identity and accountability of the participants, particularly in the light of changes to professional boundaries and the relationship between the professions, the government and the public. In this context healthcare partnerships may come to resemble the theology of the trinity which oscillates between trying to distinguish distinct persons out of a fundamental unity, or trying to establish unity from the distinct persons.

New structures

Partnership is more than just individuals working together. It is increasingly a strategic commitment which takes organisational form. Health Action Zones have created new structures for partnership. HImPs have (HAZs) established a process within which a broader field of participants can contribute to public health. PCTs create an organisational structure which allows all general practices to be involved in partnership, not just those which have previously been part of the plethora of pilots and initiatives. Partnerships may also take a variety of legal forms including, for example, independent legal partnerships, limited companies, joint ventures, charitable foundations, and community organisations (Meads *et al.* 1999: p. 30).

New partners

PCTs have not developed from the same background. They build on the relationship legacy of such different forms of primary care organisation as fundholding, multifunds, total purchasing pilots, personal medical services (PMS) pilots and many others. They also reflect differences in local politics and geography. So, for example, a trust developing from a background of a high percentage of single-handed general practices with limited experience of working together and without co-terminous health and local authority boundaries, is in a very different position to a trust in a unitary authority with a strong history of city-wide initiatives, building on the legacy of several successful primary care initiatives which have provided the opportunity for practices to work together.

Although their history is varied, primary care organisations' expectations about the range of relationships they will hold in the future are very similar – even if the form these relationships take may continue to vary widely. Table 4.1 summarises the changing pattern of relationships which consistently emerged from our work with over 50 primary care organisations during the 1997–99 period.

The relational map does, of course, depend on your viewpoint. Table 4.1 represents the views of those leading the development of PCG/Ts. If the same question is asked of those whose focus is more on the delivery of services, then a different list emerges, featuring those who are the main partners in healthcare provision. They may, however, be less attuned to the strategic requirements of organisational development and neglect these relationships. The changing number of relationships with actual or potential partners presents considerable opportunities, but will also be a difficult challenge for the NHS to manage.

Table 4.1   New primary care relationships

Pre 1998–99 general practices (3–4)	*Post 1998–99 primary care organisations (13–14)*
Intra-practice	Social services departments
Health authority	Community nursing team
Provider(s) – especially district	Clinical management groups
general hospitals	Local councils
	Local media
	Key community groups
	National monitors (e.g. NICE)
	Health authority
	Finance brokers and banks
	Pharmaceutical companies
	IM&T facilities
	NHS Direct
	Other PCG/Ts
	National Primary Care Association/ Alliance
Operational	**Strategic**

Source: Meads and Ashcroft 2000: p. 4.

Releasing the dividends – the principles
Recognising the benefits

The responses of GPs, managers and other health professionals to the changing scope of the relational map have been mixed. Some have seen the new
partnerships as an exciting opportunity to provide the kind of healthcare they have long been committed to but which has been constrained
by organisational structures. For others it has seemed a burden – another
demand on already over-pressured lives and without additional resources to
match. Developing and sustaining the relationships is merely another task; a
distraction from rather than an aid to realising the core healthcare tasks.

Effective partnerships require commitment. It is therefore important to
identify the dividends for those involved. Hudson (1998) argues per-
suasively that a presumption of altruism is an insecure basis for collaboration
and that the development of 'win–win' relationships is essential. Leadership,
learning and support are vital here. Where partnership is perceived as a duty
but not a joy, identifying realisable early benefits takes on particular importance. Where a key issue has been, for example, integrating fringe practices
which had not been part of previous inter-practice mechanisms that formed
the core of the new primary care organisation, a clear focus on the potential
of new partnerships to deal with such long-standing local issues as back
pain referrals have proved important. A focus on national priorities will not
necessarily be the most useful tactically in this regard.

The range of potential benefits from partnerships is wide, and the chapters
that follow deal with specific examples in more detail. Three groups of
benefit are worth highlighting: the potential to improve healthcare provision; financial benefits; and the organisational development dividends.
Partnerships have an important contribution to make to increasing the
accessibility of care, enabling more integrated care, improving the quality of
care and in allowing the full range of factors influencing public health to be
addressed. The same basic point applies in each case: the capacity to contribute to each of these aspects of healthcare is rarely located exclusively
within one organisation or profession. These contributions may include:
closeness of relationship to hard-to-reach groups (e.g. homeless people or
immigrant communities); the capacity to meet the different elements of the
full range of social and healthcare needs; the specialist skills to improve
quality of screening, diagnosis and treatment; or the capacity to influence the
range of social and environmental factors which may adversely affect public
health. In each of these cases there is the potential for significant dividends
for individual patients, local communities, and indeed for healthcare providers who may be more able to provide a level and quality of care beyond
that previously constrained by professional and sectoral divisions.

The financial benefits of working in partnership are closely linked to the increased trust that successful partnerships enable and the potential to access new resources. In our work with primary care organisations, the range of partners identified to provide resources has been wide, including, for example, allotment societies (with land sale proceeds), banks, pharmaceutical companies, local businesses and private healthcare providers. While these partnerships can create tensions they do allow access to additional resources without relinquishing ownership.

Sako (1997) has analysed three kinds of benefit to business performance that can arise from the presence of trust:

- it reduces transaction costs
- it allows investment to increase future returns
- it results in continuous improvement and learning.

All of these are relevant to healthcare partnerships. A context of increased trust can reduce the administrative costs of a relationship (e.g. around contracting) while retaining full accountability and appropriate financial controls. Carlisle (1999) illustrates the financial benefits from a number of industries: for example Xerox USA have estimated that the bureaucratic structures created to handle the lack of trust in their buyer/supplier relationships costs them around seven cents in the dollar. Effective healthcare partnerships should seek to reduce commissioning costs while retaining adequate processes for control and accountability. Indeed without effective processes the trust which is the key to reducing transaction costs is less likely to be maintained in the long term.

A focus on the partnership itself, and not just on transactions, provides a better context for organisational development and learning. Process improvements are usually found at the interfaces of organisational and professional relationships. The joint commitment of a partnership supports the development of all parties to increase their capacity to contribute to improvement.

Prioritising relationships

Inevitably relationships are prioritised. Whether by design or default some will get less attention than others. There is simply not enough time to develop fully all possible partnerships. It is not absolutely a zero-sum game with every investment in a new partnership requiring matching disinvestment elsewhere. New organisational forms may allow relationship management to be more widely spread but it does require a shift from individual relationships centred on GPs or service managers to more organisational relationships.

It is worth noting some consistent patterns that have tended to emerge in PCG/Ts' prioritising relationships. First there is the high priority attached to developing relationships with local authorities and social services and the absence of acute trusts. The natural first relationship for general practice, particularly in the care of vulnerable and disadvantaged groups, is with social and not secondary care. The operational relationships of working together on the frontline in the community are more important than the common legacy of a medical education. There are, however, considerable dangers if the demands of the natural, but in practice for many people often new, relationship with social services and local authorities leaves such major providers of healthcare as the acute trusts as *separate* communities and not *of* the community.

Secondly there are many new – and sometimes surprising – relationships. The task of building relationships with a local community as well as with individual patients needs new allies. These may be peculiar to specific local contexts – particularly with regard to the organisation best placed to act as finance or relationship brokers. Thirdly there are changes in the nature and importance of specific relationships. Health authorities are perhaps the strongest illustration of this as they become less active partners in the commissioning of healthcare but more the regulators of local healthcare relationships. However, as the full scope of the responsibilities commensurate with NHS trust status becomes clear, many primary care organisations have attached greater importance to their relationships with health authorities in recognition of their need for initial support in performing some of these roles. As we have seen in Chapter 2, however, these PCG/Ts have not always found a welcome for their advances.

Those who have moved most quickly to PCT status tend to have the widest range of external relationships. The demands of (and enthusiasm for) building and sustaining these many relationships has in most HMG/RF simulation exercises resulted in the neglect of internal relationships and threatened implosion. The experience of participants has been that of 'standing round a black hole facing outwards'. This is particularly a problem where the processes and responsibility for relationship management have not been developed and where relationships have not been clearly prioritised. If the burden for developing external relationships is loaded too narrowly on to a few enthusiasts, this role may be performed at the expense of developing the internal relationships needed to service fully all the commitments that flow from working in partnership with other organisations. Time is pressured and unless great care is taken it is the internal relationships which are too easily squeezed and taken for granted.

Meeting expectations

For partnerships to work it is important that both parties' expectations are met. This requires a clear definition of what these expectations are in terms of both outcomes and process. Where new relationships are forming from a weak base we have seen the importance of inclusive leadership to manage a process which gives all parties confidence that their legitimate expectations will be met, so enabling them to engage more fully and confidently in the development process.

In reviewing people's experience of relationships we have usually found that expectations are not fully realised. In some cases this is because the initial expectations are unrealistic: the initial enthusiasm for new forms of inter-professional working in one PMS pilot, for example, meant that the difficulties were underestimated. In other cases it will be because expectations take time to be realised – relationships take time to mature and there are few short cuts in this process. There will also be cases where remedial action is needed if the intended dividends are to be realised.

A unifying focus

Partnerships need a strong unifying focus. While shared accountability to the requirements of central objectives provides a helpful context for PCTs this is rarely sufficient to cement local partnerships, particularly if the relationships are immature or strained. At an operational level a strong shared commitment to a client group can be a powerful force: while this may produce pockets of effective collaboration it may not be enough for organisation-wide partnerships.

A common 'enemy' often helps cement partnerships. Overspending acute trusts have often fulfilled this role for primary care organisations, although their response to this 'enemy' can vary widely. On the one hand there is the option of primary care organisations collaborating to compete for resources more effectively. Here the dividend of partnership is to increase the resources made available to primary care. In some cities we have visited there has been a concern to extend the partnership to include the acute trust. Working with the acute trust was felt to offer more options for dealing with long-standing resource problems, and also to provide a better context for developing ways in which the acute trust could support more accessible provision of specialist services to local communities.

Accepting change and managing the process

Effective partnerships will not be ossified. They are likely to be characterised by growth, change and evolution and therefore require a willingness to embrace change. This has implications for PCTs' strategic processes, which will need to become more flexible and emergent, and also for the basis of individual, professional and organisational security. The processes of organisational development and strategy, informed by review, with clear milestones to ensure that partnership relationships are in fact supporting the achievement of the desired outcomes, are the issues to which we now turn.

Releasing the dividends – the processes

All aspects of healthcare management and delivery have a contribution to make to releasing the dividends of partnerships. Here we focus on three aspects: strategy, development and review. These are interrelated since a relational strategy must be informed by some assessments of the relationships that are in place. We have seen in PCGs too many strategies which presume a nature and quality of relationship which do not in fact exist. For relationships, in particular, it is important to maintain the link between review and development. Too often performance management can neglect relationships or even create perverse relationship-inhibiting incentives. The value of reviewing relationships should not be seen purely in terms of enabling control, but rather in its capacity to support development which, in the context of a learning organisation, enables what Senge (1990) has termed 'personal mastery'. Development also feeds back into strategy for it is often in the course of joint development work that strategy emerges. We have also seen that the process of working together in PCG/Ts to develop joint strategies, particularly on such issues as public health, can provide significant development opportunities.

Key questions

No two relationships are the same: this is as true for organisational relationships as it is for interpersonal relationships. There is, therefore, no one-size-fits-all model of NHS partnerships. Whatever the particular nature of a partnership, there are a range of processes for developing and managing the partnership to help ensure that the potential dividends of that partnership are realised. The development of a partnership involves a number of stages (*see* Table 4.2) although not always as a simple sequential process. At each of these stages there are a number of critical questions to be asked.

Table 4.2   Stages of partnership development

Selection	Design	Negotiation	Building	Improvement	(Rescue)
Is this the right partner?	What is a 'good' relationship?	How will it operate?	What are the foundations?	What are the processes for review?	How are problems identified and resolved?
Screening for relational 'fit'	Agreeing the outcomes	Aligning expectations	Putting the preconditions in place	Assessing strengths and weaknesses	Identifying the causal factors

Partnerships are not always chosen – the partnership may be a statutory duty or there may be no alternative partners. In these cases selection is not so much about choosing but recognising at the outset whether there is a natural fit or whether there are, for example, significantly divergent objectives which will need to be acknowledged or resolved.

Each PCG/T will need to answer the question as to what they mean by a 'good' relationship in the context of each partnership. This may be, in part, a functional definition with different outcomes being prioritised, but will also reflect different preferences and priorities for the style of the relationship. If they are trying to create different kinds of relationship then the dividends of that partnership are less likely to be fully realised. This is not to say that all parties should hold exactly the same understanding, but rather where there are differences these should either be discussed so that a consensus is reached, or acknowledged and accommodated so that the needs of each party to the relationship are met.

A simple way of exploring these issues is to brainstorm the possible outcomes. Imagine that you have 100 points to allocate across the outcomes raised. Compare your allocation with your counterparts and discuss the reasons for different priorities. An example of such a discussion is given in Table 4.3.

In negotiating the development of a new (or the new stage of a) partnership relationship it is important to clarify expectations. Given the multi-professional profile of PCG/Ts, divergent views here are likely to cause friction and frustration later so it is worth investing time up front to align expectations and challenge false assumptions. This is particularly important where organisations are not used to working together and where the relationship is complicated by different professional and organisational cultures. It is all too easy to assume that others will work in the same way to which you are accustomed. If this process is done thoroughly it can

Table 4.3 A 'good' relationship ...

Requires little change	Encourages and supports change
Is low risk:	Brings in new:
• politically	• skills
• financially	• resources
• personally	• ideas
• clinically	• opportunities
Fosters innovation	Is high trust
Has low administrative costs	Is robust when difficulties emerge
Offers choice and flexibility	Is personally satisfying
Requires limited investment	Is worth considerable investment
Enhances relationships with:	Improves:
• individual patients	• quality of care
• the local community	• accessibility of care
• other partners	• integration of care
	• choice of care

also be used to frame the performance standards for the relationship and provide a benchmark for subsequent review.

Relationships, no less than other areas of healthcare activity, need to be monitored and managed for maximum effectiveness. Yet too often performance management ignores the relationships that underpin performance, and can even create perverse, relationship-destroying incentives. Ensuring that there are appropriate processes for reviewing partnerships is important and these require their own methods. The tools for financial control or clinical trials do not provide the best basis for evaluating relationships and retaining the organic relationship between development and performance management which is so important. Reviews should also be able to identify the range of causal factors which may influence the relationship. These indicate the areas where specific actions may help to release the dividends of partnership. They may be people factors concerning, for example, skills, structural factors or working practices.

A framework for review

A framework we have found useful in working with many primary care organisations is to look at preconditions for relationships. These are a set of necessary but not sufficient conditions for effective relationships (however defined) to develop. This framework, developed by the Relationships Foundation (Schluter and Lee 1993) includes five elements (*see* Table 4.4).

Table 4.4   A framework for review

Precondition	*Description*
Directness	**Quality of the communication process**
Medium of communication	Right medium to maximise amount/quality of Information exchange
Access and responsiveness	Direct communication avoiding delay and Misunderstandings
Style/skills	Communication characterised by listening, openness and honesty
Continuity	**Shared time over time**
Amount/regularity of contact	Investment of time and sufficiency of contact in the relationship
Length/stability	Consistency in the relationship, continuing commitment to it
Managing change	Maintaining the continuity of the relationship through change
Multiplexity	**Breadth of knowledge**
Organisation/ department	Work constraints and opportunities of the other, the issues they face
Task/function	Understanding of role and the skills and experience the other brings
Personal understanding	Informal contact, knowledge of personal interests, goals and values
Parity	**Use and abuse of power**
Participation	Involvement in decision making within the relationship
Fair benefits	Arrangements that represent fair distribution of risk and reward
Fair conduct	Application of standards, treating people with respect and integrity
Commonality	**Valuing similarity and difference**
Shared objectives	Common view of objectives, priorities and the means of achieving them
Common culture	Way of working reflects understanding of operating environment
Positive diversity	Recognition of different views, valuing new perspectives

Directness

Directness influences the quality of communication in the relationship. The medium of communication affects the amount and quality of information exchanged. Face-to-face communication, for example, allows non-verbal signals to be picked up and immediate responses to be made, so enabling better understanding. It is perhaps of particular importance around difficult or particularly important issues. It is, however, resource intensive so it is important to ensure that the right medium is used at the right time.

The channel of communication influences both the quality and efficiency of information exchange. Both can be reduced if channels are blocked or if information and decisions are too often received secondhand, via messages or through several levels of bureaucracy. Accessibility and responsiveness are key issues here. Communication style and skills are also significant. The structure of the communication must be complemented by the right behaviour. For instance, a lack of openness can impede trust and undermine partnership. A cycle operates here: openness can create trust, and trust can encourage openness, but a downward spiral of decreased trust and impaired communication can also develop.

This aspect of the relationship is often tested in commissioning and strategic processes. At its worst, particularly, in the context of new and difficult relationships, direct communication has been too threatening and parallel development processes have had to be run in order to establish a minimum baseline of commonality to sustain open communication. Unvoiced (or unheeded) concerns and (suspected) hidden agendas still distort consultation processes. Even in mature and successful relationships it has been difficult for PCG/Ts and health authorities to sustain directness in the midst of commissioning processes and the associated demands for information (Meads *et al.* 1999).

Continuity

A lack of continuity has been a common recent NHS experience. Although time, which can be seen as the currency of relationships, has been pressured for most people their principal concern has not been around the amount of contact. Rather it has been around the legacy of change and the impact of staff turnover.

The length and stability of the relationship over time creates the opportunity for individual rapport and improved mutual understanding to develop, as well as providing a context for long-term issues to be addressed at an organisational level. Where staff turnover is high – as we have found in many parts of the local NHS in London – locking in the benefits of individual and informal relationships to create an organisational history and overview of the relationship is often important. Managing change in the relationship is important if such benefits of change, such as career progression and bringing in new people, are to be achieved without undermining the quality and effectiveness of existing relationships.

Multiplexity

Multiplexity looks at the breadth of the relationship. This can enhance mutual understanding and enable a broader appreciation of the range of skills and experience that individuals or organisations can contribute. It helps avoid strategies which ignore the realities of the underlying relationships and may open up new opportunities that arise from unsuspected common ground or unrecognised resources. Knowledge of a counterpart's organisation or department is important to appreciate the constraints under which they work, to identify shared objectives and to develop appropriate ways of joint working. Knowledge of role or skills is important for the effectiveness of joint work and helps avoid flawed assumptions or misunderstandings, missed opportunities or sub-optimal resource utilisation. Knowledge of the person (such as his or her interests or values) can strengthen the relationship and aid its management.

This is often an uncertain dimension of healthcare relationships. We have found it is often evident, for example, in the mutual ignorance of NHS and local authority staff about each others' organisations. This applies, particularly, to PCG/Ts with limited histories of corporate working and SSD collaboration. Failure to understand different decision-making processes, structures, and ways of working were also seen as major problems in partnership working around HImPs. For the new strategic relationships there is much groundwork yet to be done.

Parity

At times it is hard to find anyone who believes they have power in an NHS relationship. Parity does not mean equality in a relationship. Authority, influence or rewards in a relationship may rightly vary, although it is important that differentials are accepted and not abused. It is rarely a simple picture, for there are many different kinds of power (financial control, regulatory or sapiential authority, political influence, control of delivery, or exit and veto rights) in a relationship, and different parties in a relationship are likely to have different kinds of power.

Parity requires, and is fostered by, participation and involvement which ensures that people have some real say in decisions which affect their work. Lack of participation may mean that strategic objectives are not owned, may reduce morale and stifle innovation. Inadequate influence in a relationship with respect to tasks or responsibilities is a frequent source of frustration.

The fairness of benefits in a relationship can engender co-operation and foster commitment to a relationship from which both parties can benefit. Fair conduct in the relationship is necessary for trust and respect. This is often cited by people whose experience of inter-professional relationships has not always been characterised by mutual respect as a major obstacle to effective collaboration. Double standards, prejudice and favouritism are extremely corrosive. The shortfalls on parity are a major challenge for PCG/Ts to address in creating the kinds of adult–adult relationships referred to by PCT chief executives in Chapter 2 as key long-term objectives.

Commonality

Commonality enables individuals and organisations to work together towards shared goals. While tensions can be creative, and there may be differences in roles and responsibilities, if these are not set in the context of some shared objectives and understanding, then the likelihood of per-formance-hindering conflict may be increased. Common objectives provide the basis for working together. Without real, shared, defined objectives (as opposed to generalised goals) organisations or teams may end up pulling in different directions or come into conflict over priorities. Agreement over the means of achieving goals may be as important as agreement about the goals themselves. The process by which agreement on objectives is reached is important in building commonality. Many of the PCG strategic processes we have witnessed have been hampered by differing views of health (and local health priorities) as well as competing organisational interests.

Shared culture reduces the risk of misunderstandings, difficulty in artic-ulating shared objectives and the lack of a shared basis for resolving differ-ences of opinion. This applies to both professional and organisational cultures. A sense of common identity, of ultimately being in the same boat, can reflect the strength of the relationship as well as providing a basis for its development. This may be expressed through establishing some com-mon culture or through developing working practices which take account of different cultures rather than just working round them or simply ignoring them. Commonality does not require uniformity. Differences can add value to a relationship though it is important that they are seen as enriching the relationship and not just as obstacles to be overcome. The way in which disagreements are handled is also important: their resolution can strengthen commonality or may only seek to reinforce the differences. Different professional and organisational cultures in the contemporary NHS have been a frequent problem, creating misunderstanding and mistrust, as well as competing interests. PCTs, as broad churches, offer new opportunities to respond positively to these dilemmas.

Relational mapping

Working with primary care organisations around this framework has revealed many issues which limit the extent to which the full dividends of partnership are being realised. First there are many relationships where the pre-conditions are simply not in place. Using the relational mapping tool (*see* Table 4.5) there are many low scores. A PCG in the South West, for example, scored less than 50% in its relationships with social services and the public. District councils, the local media, education agencies and voluntary organisations did not reach even these scores, even though they were the relationships identified by the PCG as crucial to legitimising their future decision making (Meads and Ashcroft 2000: p. 33).

Relational mapping provides a simple exercise which brings together review and development. The strategic process of identifying key relationships, and jointly reflecting on high-level indicators of their nature and quality, is a revealing process. Table 4.5 is a general example. We have often used this in the context of a future scenario which focuses attention on the new relationships to be developed, and also the changing requirements of these relationships as components of a wider health strategy. The process of identifying and prioritising relationships is revealing (the list in Table 4.1 comes from using this approach). It can highlight development needs, and also the different contributions to a partnership.

The way ahead

Strategy

Realising the dividends of new partnerships is, in part, a strategic issue. The importance of these partnerships also means that the NHS will need to approach strategy in new ways. Too narrow a focus on planning and structures will not help chart a way through the dynamic landscape of healthcare relationships. Rather, strategy must be a relational process which: identifies the right partners; is participative and inclusive; is efficient and effective; and which is authentically emergent from the process, flexible and responsive.

Table 4.5 Relational mapping

You are a newly formed PCT. Bearing in mind both your immediate and long-term responsibilities, identify and agree the five relationships which are most important to maintain or develop (these may be either within the PCT or with other organisations, groups or individuals).

For each of these relationships rate their relative strengths and weaknesses for each relational precondition on a 1–5 scale (5 = high).

Discuss the reasons for any notable areas of strength or weakness. Suggest one or two actions for strengthening the weakest aspects of each of these relationships.

Relationship *Relational pre-conditions*

	Directness	**Continuity**	**Multiplexity**	**Parity**	**Commonality**
e.g. Between member practices	4	3	3	2 Identify areas for increased participation by 'fringe' practices	2
1					
2					
3					
4					
5					

Discussion questions:
- Which relationships have been selected?
  - Are people agreed? If not, why not?
  - What are the different reasons for selection? The strategic importance of the relationship? Because delivery will not happen without them? Because of the importance of the client group they represent?
  - Would the same relationships be selected in five years' time? Which become more or less important? How will activities and time allocation change to reflect this? How are relationships of future importance being cultivated?
- Which relationships are stronger or weaker?
  - Do people agree on scores? If not does this reflect their different experience? Or different weighting attached to different aspects of each dimension?
  - Which of the relationships are notably strong or weak compared to the others? Do they feel the best or the worst? What kind of relationships are they, e.g. operational or strategic; new or old; inter-organisational or inter-professional?
  - What are the likely consequences of any weakness in these relationships? How can these be mitigated?
- Do any dimensions of the relationships tend to be weaker or stronger?
  - If so, what are the reasons for this? Does this reflect generic pressures on healthcare relationships (e.g. cultural or structural issues)?
  - What are the consequences of weaknesses in these aspects of the relationships? How can they be ameliorated?

Strategic partnerships

Strategy is, accordingly for PCTs, about seeking the right relationships, and working with potential partners to encourage future fit. For businesses the key to competitive advantage is seen in 'building relationships with customers, suppliers and employees that are exceptionally hard for competitors to duplicate' (Waterman 1994: p. 170). So, too, for healthcare organisations: the best contribution to healthcare will arise from a strategy which develops the right kind of relationships with the right partners who can contribute to that process.

Participative and inclusive strategy

Harnessing the contributions of partners, and so realising the dividends of partnership, requires involvement. In the context of multi-sectoral and multi-agency approaches to delivering healthcare the knowledge base and resources are diffuse. Accessing this knowledge and ensuring the ownership and commitment that is required to make progress requires higher degrees of involvement. Yet, in many of the workshops we have run, those who have most to contribute can often be the last to speak. In one London district, for example, in an illuminating exercise where 12 primary care professionals took it in turns to chair a mock PCG meeting and invite contributions from each other with a view to improving local health, it was the local optometrist and community pharmacist who seemed to have the most to offer, but they were only chosen to speak at the ninth and tenth times of asking (Meads and Ashcroft 2000: p. 41). Real participation fosters commitment and ensures that the partnership strategy realistically reflects the relational resources. This may involve systematic dialogue with the network of stakeholder relationships. Such an approach can be supported by social audits (*see*, for example, Wheeler and Sillanpaa 1997) to ensure that there is a sustained cycle of inclusion.

Efficient, effective and emergent

There is always the danger in the closed world of some primary care organisations that what may feel like a good relationship can be inefficient, ineffective, cosy, collusive and complacent. Conversely, relationships which can appear to be under considerable strain may be in fact be the most robust and healthy. An inclusive strategy is not a recipe for talking shops; inclusion is a style of leadership not a substitute for it.

The environment of healthcare relationships is always changing. Relationships cannot easily be controlled (locally or centrally) and attempting to do so is often counterproductive. Strategy must therefore be responsive to this changing environment. This is not a recipe for short-termism. Rather it is about creating organisations and strategic processes which can cope with change and continually readjust strategies to achieve their long-term aims.

The extent of the cultural change and challenge this implies should not be underestimated. Modern healthcare partnerships will need continually to live with change. Strategy involves continually readjusting to the changing local health economy. The old securities (if, in fact, they ever existed) of control and stability must be, in part, exchanged for the security that comes from robust partnerships, community legitimacy and acknowledged success and quality in delivery. Indeed this security is one of the dividends of new partnerships – relationships can endure through change in a way that structures do not.

This chapter reaches its close with an example of what a relational strategy might look like. This was developed in the course of a simulation as part of a Health Education Authority funded programme to look at how primary care organisations could improve public health as well as deliver healthcare (Meads *et al.* 1999). The 'Franchised Company' was one of the four organisational types identified as part of the project. Its detailed profile was set out earlier in Chapter 2. Although there are currently few organisational developments with a comprehensive approach to assuming a franchised responsibility for the local population's health and healthcare, this was the aspiration for many of the districts where we have worked. It is a model for tomorrow's PCTs of the real dividends to be derived from 'new' partnerships.

> *The Franchised Company*
> The Franchised Company has the most comprehensive health strategy of the four organisational types (defined in the HEA programme). Its mission is to improve the health and wellbeing of the population and to reduce health inequalities and social exclusion. This language is important at this level because it incorporates the roles (and expectations) of both the Department of Health and local government, focusing on 'inequalities' as a joint and shared priority. It means the organisations need to engage in a bottom-up approach to assessing needs and selecting priorities and therefore to questioning 'old priorities'. The actual process of engaging communities is paramount. It is based on a range of methods which recognise the natural communities which make up the population and can include whole systems approaches, focus groups and citizens' juries.

Its specific strategies for priority areas span the full continuum of needs of population groups to improve their health and well-being, that is health services, local government services and community development. For example, plans for older people cover hip replacements, community safety, transport, housing, heating and social networks.

Its planning is based on the totality of NHS and local government resources and expenditure for the PCG population, plus an awareness of the possible resources available in other sectors. It uses sophisticated programme planning techniques, for example health impact assessment analysis, to enable alternative investment strategies to be tested. All stakeholders, including communities, participate in debates about investment and rationing decisions. There is an increased awareness and ownership of resource consequences of investment choices. Balanced judgements that recognise the need to meet certain national standards and requirements as well as respond to local priorities characterise this level, as do different styles of service provision. The design and delivery of services based on new ways of involving families, individuals and communities include delegated budgets to communities, and advocacy for isolated/vulnerable groups; and support to an infrastructure of community groups.

Concerned with ensuring that wider policies and strategies operate to promote the health and wellbeing of the local communities and address inequalities, this organisation tests the boundaries of regulations and seeks freedoms to operate in more integrated and flexible ways. It recognises the need to ensure that quality standards and effective practice are adopted, for example via the National Institute for Clinical Excellence, and that standards are universally available to socially excluded groups (Meads *et al.* 1999).

References

Carlisle J (1999) *Co-operation Works … But it's Hard Work.* John Carlisle Partnerships, Sheffield.

Hudson R (1998) *Primary Care and Social Care.* Nuffield Institute, Leeds.

Meads G and Ashcroft J (2000) *Relationships in the NHS: bridging the gap.* Royal Society of Medicine Press, London.

Meads G, Killoran A, Ashcroft J and Cornish Y (1999) *Mixing Oil and Water.* HEA Publications, London.

Sako M (1997) Does trust improve business performance? In: C Lane and R Beckmann (eds) *Trust Within and Between Organisations*. Oxford University Press, Oxford.

Schulter M and Lee D (1993) *The 'R' Factor*. Hodder and Stoughton, London.

Secretary of State for Health (1997) *The New NHS: modern, dependable*. Department of Health, London.

Senge P (1990) *The Fifth Discipline: the art and science of a learning organisation*. Century, London.

Waterman R (1994) *The Frontiers of Excellence: learning from companies that put people first*. Nicholas Brearley Publishing, London.

Wheeler D and Sillanpaa M (1997) *The Stakeholder Corporation*. Pitman Publishing, London.

CHAPTER 5

Owning up to the public health agenda

Yvonne Cornish

No injustice is greater than the inequalities in health which scar our nation.[1]

Walking upstream

One of the key themes running through health policy, at all levels, is that to improve the health of individuals, communities and populations, we need to do much more than provide high quality, accessible and appropriate services. We also need to move towards what is sometimes called 'upstream thinking'.

This notion of 'upstream thinking' comes from a tale often told in public health circles, which equates health workers to life-savers standing beside a fast-flowing river:

> Every so often, a drowning person is swept alongside. The life-saver dives in to the rescue, retrieves 'the patient' and resuscitates them. Just as they have finished, another casualty appears alongside. So busy and involved are the life-savers in all of this rescue work that they have no time to walk upstream and see why it is that so many people are falling into the river. (Ashton and Seymour 1988)

Recognition of the need to 'walk upstream' to improve health, rather than concentrating entirely on treatment and care of the sick, dates back to antiquity. According to legend, the ancient Greeks were watched over by the goddess Hygeia. This deity, whose name derives from an abstract word meaning 'health', symbolised the belief that good health could be achieved

---

[1] *NHS Plan* 2000: 13.1

by living wisely. From around the fifth century BC onwards, the cult of Hygeia was gradually replaced by that of Asclepius, the god of healing. As the first physician in Greek mythology, Asclepius achieved fame through the practice of surgery and the curative use of plants. But Hygeia did not disappear entirely. In much representation, Asclepius is accompanied by two daughters – on his right Hygeia, and on his left her sister Panakeia (Dubos 1984).

Dubos argues that: 'The myths of Hygeia and Asclepius symbolise the never-ending oscillation' between preventative and curative approaches to illness and disease. The tension between these two approaches is still clearly evident today, with ongoing debates around the relative importance of prevention versus treatment in the improvement of health. These debates are not merely of academic interest. They continue to underpin decision making and resource allocation at all levels of policy and practice, and therefore have considerable implications for the future development and delivery of primary care.

'Saving Lives' – the policy challenge

'Upstream thinking' is at the forefront of the health strategy *Saving Lives: our healthier nation* (Secretary of State 1999). This White Paper sets out a comprehensive approach to the task of improving the health of individuals and communities. The two main goals of *Saving Lives: our healthier nation* are by now familiar to most of us. They are, of course:

- to improve the health of the population as a whole by increasing the length of people's lives and the number of years which people spend free from illness
- to improve the health of the worst off in society and to narrow the health gap.

This health strategy draws on the wealth of evidence from the social, behavioural and biological sciences which has demonstrated that improvements in health are influenced as much by social, economic and environmental factors as by genetic predisposition, lifestyle or individual behaviour. As such, it acknowledges that policy and practice aimed at improving health and reducing the 'burden of disease' will need to be broad-based, collaborative, and informed by multi-disciplinary approaches.

Health is determined by more than health services – and health policy is at last recognising this. In moving from a relatively narrow focus on medical treatment and care to a much broader concern with *any* policy which affects health, the current government argues that health is everyone's responsibility. As a result, there is a strong emphasis across government on the need for 'joined-up' policy making at all levels, supported by (and in support of) partnership working across public sector organisations to deliver shared public health goals.

What does this mean for primary care?

How will the new PCGs and PCTs engage with this agenda? The goals set out in *Saving Lives* are reflected in the Department of Health guidance on the functions of PCG/Ts. For example, *Primary Care Groups: delivering the agenda* (NHS Executive 1998a), set out the three main functions of the new primary care organisations as being to:

- improve the health of, and address health inequalities in, their community
- develop primary and community health services across their area
- commission secondary care services appropriate to patients' needs.

PCTs will have similar responsibilities for improving health and addressing inequalities, as well as for delivering effective services (Box 5.1).

Box 5.1   Improving the health of the community – the role of PCTs

PCTs will take on responsibility for improving the health of their community and addressing local health inequalities. They will need to ensure that a range of services are available for their population which are delivered to a consistently high quality and are efficient and effective. In meeting these requirements they will need to engage with and involve patients, carers and local partner organisations. The needs of their community might be met more effectively through partnership working or development and support of non-health service provision.

Source: NHSE 1999

However, PCTs will have access to a wider range of skills and expertise at executive level than PCGs, and greater flexibilities to support joint working – including the flexibility for NHS and local authorities to delegate their health improvement-related functions to each other and to pool budgets for specific services, including services which might improve health or reduce inequalities in the health of their local communities.

Improving health – the partnership challenge

One of the key partnerships needed to deliver health improvement at a local level will clearly be the partnership between public health and primary care. However, recognition of the need for public health and primary care to work more closely together is not new. Like the 'new public health' (*see below*) it has its roots in the World Health Organization's 'Health for All' strategy, which highlighted the need to strengthen primary healthcare and to refocus services on the promotion of health and prevention of disease (WHO 1978). It has also been advocated by pioneering general practitioners such as Julian Tudor Hart, who argued for a 'new kind of doctor', who, in addition to being responsible for personal care, would provide a neighbourhood public health function – identifying unmet health needs, running screening programmes and actively promoting the health of local communities (Tudor Hart 1984). An 'upstream' approach was even (to some extent) enshrined in the Thatcher government's policy agenda for developing primary care services. It was *Promoting Better Health* (DHSS 1987) and the 1990 GP contract, after all, which introduced routine health checks for specific sectors of the population, targets for childhood immuni-sation and cervical cytology, and sessional fees for health promotion clinics in primary care (Moon and North 2000).

However, the recent policy focus, which takes a multi-dimensional view of health and how it can be improved, combined with a recognition of the need to tackle the wider social and economic determinants of ill-health, has given the need for an 'upstream' approach much greater emphasis. Further-more, the task key players are being given is clearly a shared one. Whilst policies that are set out as 'joined up' at the level of central government may appear fragmented at a grass roots level, the emphasis on working in partnership enables all the stakeholders to bring the fragments together. As one participant, reflecting on recent government health policy during a seminar run by members of the Health Management Group, remarked:

> ... it's a jigsaw puzzle ... but I'm not sure who it is going to be given to. We seem to each be being given a different piece ... perhaps the government wants us to do it together? (GP participant at a workshop for *Mixing Oil and Water*, Meads *et al.* 1999)

Yet, as Graham Winyard asks in his forward to the aptly-named report on public health and primary care *Shared Contribution, Shared Benefits*, 'The question is how primary care and public health working together can achieve these goals more effectively than if they work separately' (NHSE 1998b). In other words, how can they form the kind of partnership that will deliver improvements in the health of their local communities, and reduce inequalities in health status?

In Chapter 4, John Ashcroft sets out some of the key principles for effective partnership working. To what extent might these principles apply to public health and primary care? For example, do the key players recognise the benefits that might accrue from the partnership? Do they have the potential to meet each other's expectations? Is there a strong and unifying focus to cement their partnership? The next section of this chapter will examine some of these questions in more depth, by looking at some of the professional history each of the partners brings to the relationship. The final section will return to the main theme of this book, and explore the considerable opportunities for transferable learning that are likely to emerge as PCTs move towards becoming public health organisations.

The 'science and art' of public health

Public health has been defined as 'the science and art of preventing disease, prolonging life, and promoting health, through the organised efforts of society' (Acheson 1988). However, as the history of public health shows, ideas about how this should be achieved have not only changed over time — but continue to underpin current debates around health improvement.

Moreover, 'public health', like 'primary care' (*see below*), is also understood to mean a number of different things. At its broadest, it simply means 'the health of the public' — but it is also used to describe a body of knowledge, a professional group, a department within the health authority, or a 'function' within (and beyond) the NHS. A recent report on public health and primary care (Taylor *et al.* 1998) noted 'a crucial distinction between public health as a resource, and public health as action' which was mirrored in their research fieldwork:

> Health professionals understood 'public health' as information about the patterns of disease and standards of treatment and services. Lay people saw the term itself as referring to things like clean drains or head lice. They did not immediately see their health-based community activities as being part of a public health agenda … (*ibid.* pp. 56–57)

So, where do these different understandings and expectations come from? To understand this, we need to take a brief look at the history of public health.

From sanitary reform to public health medicine

The modern public health movement has its origins in the nineteenth century. Industrialisation and the rapid growth of cities were accompanied by high levels of infectious diseases, and the health impact of the physical environment was increasingly recognised and documented. Urban poverty, overcrowding, poor housing conditions, contaminated water supplies and 'bad air' were major concerns, and local authorities in many towns and cities appointed Medical Officers of Health to advise them on dealing with these problems. Interventions to improve health have been described as 'sanitary reform' in that they predominantly took the form of large-scale civil engineering projects, such as the installation of sewage systems and the provision of clean drinking water.

Towards the end of the nineteenth century, and throughout the early twentieth century, as the mechanisms for the transmission of infectious diseases became better understood, interventions to prevent them took a more individualistic turn. There was a greater emphasis on personal prevention (through increasing the resistance of the individual) than on social or environmental change (reducing the source of infection). Public health interventions during this period included the introduction of immunisation programmes, advice on personal hygiene, and more general health education (in the form of providing information on the causes of diseases, and how they could be prevented). Community health services were also developed in an attempt to reduce the continuing high levels of infant and child mortality, and to improve the health of school-aged children.

From the 1930s onwards, as therapeutic interventions became increasingly successful and curative approaches to health improvement became more dominant, public health practice was further weakened. When the NHS was established, public health initially remained in local government, though gradually it became professionally separated from environmental health and other emerging specialist roles, such as social work and health visiting. In the early 1970s, with the establishment of social services departments in local government, public health and community medicine finally moved into the NHS – leaving responsibility for environmental health in local government, where it has remained ever since.

The 'new public health' and 'Health for All'

Around this time, however, a more integrated approach to health improvement began to re-emerge. This was driven by a number of factors, including a growing recognition that neither curative medicine, nor an individualistic approach to disease prevention, had succeeded in reducing inequalities in health status, or in reducing the burden of preventable disease. This approach, which was soon to become known as the 'new public health', followed publication of the Lalond Report (1974) in Canada, which restated the importance of taking a multi-dimensional approach to improving health. The 'new public health' was further influenced by the World Health Organization's resolution in 1977, that the main social goal of the WHO and participating governments should be 'the attainment, by all the people of the world, by the year 2000, of a level of health that will permit them to lead a socially and economically productive life' (WHO 1978).

'Health for All 2000' as it became known (now HFA 2001) was then the subject of regional interpretation and target-setting (WHO 1985). In 1980, the HFA European targets were underpinned by the following key features:

- the reorientation of services
- a move towards a more holistic view of health
- recognition of the social and environmental influences on health
- the importance of health education in promoting healthy lifestyles
- the aim to reduce inequalities in health.

Whilst HFA approaches and targets were taken up into local policy-making in many areas (for example, in the 'Healthy Cities' move-ment), and informed the development of theory and practice in health promotion, it was some time before the UK Government developed a health strategy for England. (*See The Health of the Nation: a strategy for England* 1992.)

Public health and health service reform

Meanwhile, public health practice in the NHS became very much locked into the NHS reforms of the early 1990s. The Acheson review, *Public Health in England* (Acheson 1988), which had been set up in response to two major outbreaks of infectious diseases and a growing concern about HIV and AIDS, considerably strengthened the role of public health within health authorities. It also led to the revival of Annual Public Health Reports, which were to be an independent statement, by the Director of Public Health, on the health needs and health status of the local population. HC 1988/064, the Health Circular which implemented the Acheson report, made public health central to the role of health authorities (Box 5.2) (Department of Health 1988).

These responsibilities were reinforced by *Working for Patients* (Depart-ment of Health 1990) which outlined the new role of health authorities as 'ensuring the health needs of the population for which they are responsible

---

Box 5.2   Health of the population – responsibilities of health
authorities

- Review regularly the health of the population
- Define policy aims and set objectives to deal with any problems
- Relate decisions on resource allocation to their impact on health
- Monitor and evaluate progress towards their objectives
- Arrange for the surveillance, prevention, treatment and control of
  communicable diseases

Source: Department of Health 1988/064

---

are met; that there are effective services for the prevention and control of
diseases and the promotion of health; that their population has access to a
comprehensive range of high quality, value-for-money services; and on
setting targets for and monitoring ... performance ...'.

Public health and health promotion

As the internal market developed, two things happened which worked
against the maintenance of an integrated approach to public health. The
first was that public health staff (especially public health doctors) were
increasingly occupied supporting the purchasing function within the health
authority. Their work on health needs assessment and service evaluation
often took priority over inter-sectoral working with local government and
the wider community on the economic and social determinants of health,
and public health physicians were frequently called upon to support commissioning managers in difficult negotiations with clinicians over contracting issues (Cornish, unpublished thesis).

The second factor was the uncertainty over the role of health promotion. At the inception of the internal market, health promotion departments
were in general located within, or managerially subsumed under, public
health departments. Whilst some health authorities continued this arrange-
ment, others redefined health promotion as a provider activity, and moved it
into a community trust. As a result, public health and health promotion have
come to be seen as largely different tasks, underpinned by different models of
health, as highlighted in the model developed by Scott Samuel (Figure 5.1).

There are some early indications that, with the advent of PCG/Ts, this
model may now be being superseded. For example, public health and health
promotion staff taking part in a recent training event in South London
argued that the two circles in this model were moving closer together, and

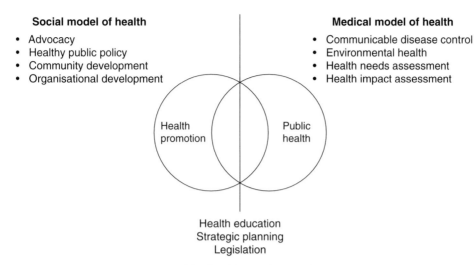

Social model of health

- Advocacy
- Healthy public policy
- Community development
- Organisational development

Medical model of health

- Communicable disease control
- Environmental health
- Health needs assessment
- Health impact assessment

Health promotion

Public health

Health education
Strategic planning
Legislation

Figure 5.1   Scott Samuel's model of public health and health promotion.
Source: Black 1999.

that there was some sharing or even exchanging of areas of responsibility. However, it is not clear how extensive this change might be. Also, the role of the local authority in health improvement is not included in Scott Samuel's model, and this now clearly needs to be taken into account.

Following a research review into the implementation of *The Health of the Nation* in North Thames (Cornish, Russell *et al.* 1997), two of the review team undertook further analysis of the qualitative data gathered for the project, and found that the key players in the implementation process for this health strategy were working with different conceptual models of health, and therefore had different views on what could, or should, be done to bring about health improvement (*see* Figure 5.2) (Cornish and Russell 1998).

As PCTs will discover, these different understandings of the health improvement task frequently lead to the adoption of different styles of working, and make it difficult to agree shared priorities for action. Whilst there was evidence that key players in successful partnerships had developed an understanding of each other's priorities, timetables, budgetary and financial constraints, and even of each other's organisational cultures, a shared understanding of what constitutes health, and how it could be improved, was more elusive – and this has implications for the development of a sense of 'common purpose'. If, as we found, this lack of a shared understanding of health is an issue for public health and health promotion staff working within and across health and local authorities, we could reasonably anticipate that it could be an issue which will need addressing when public health and health promotion professionals work with colleagues in primary care, and for primary care partnerships with local authorities.

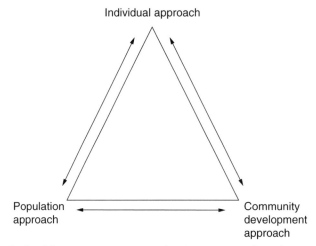

Figure 5.2 The health improvement triangle. *Source*: Cornish and Russell 1998.

Primary care – defining diversity

The history of primary care is also a history of changing ideas and approaches, and, like public health, echoes of earlier forms continue to exist alongside recent developments. 'Official' definitions vary considerably, depending on the source. Two contrasting examples, derived from an early project on public health and primary care undertaken by the Regional Directors of Public Health Group (Cornish and Griffiths 1993) are given in Box 5.3.

Box 5.3   Competing definitions of primary care

... a network of service that covers the whole spectrum of health and social care: prevention for the young and well, treatment of acute and chronic illness, rehabilitation, respite care, residential care, support at home for patients who are frail, elderly, disabled and acutely or chronically ill, and terminal care. (King's Fund)

'Primary' is used widely to include any health professional whose professional qualification is in healthcare, whose professional qualification is recognised by a statutory council approved by Parliament, who sees clients/patients direct without any referral from another health professional, or who

---

> works within a primary medical or nursing care organisation that offers patients open access ... 'Primary care' is taken to mean dentists (General Dental Practitioners), pharmacists, and opticians. (Royal College of General Practitioners.)
> *Source*: Cornish and Griffiths 1993

So, like public health, primary care is on some occasions taken to mean a group of professionals, and on others to refer to the services they provide. In addition, primary care is also often used interchangeably with general practice, though in fact general practice is only one part of a comprehensive primary care service, which is currently undergoing a period of rapid change. This change is more than organisational – that is, it is not simply a change from individual practice to PCG and then on to PCT. It is also, as Meads has argued, a change from primary medical care (epitomised by a clinically-orientated personal physician, who responds to the demands of his registered list, and acts as 'gatekeeper' to secondary care), through primary managed care (in which the primary care team works to group targets, protocols and standards on an inter-professional basis, thereby managing the demand for secondary care), to primary healthcare (which is population-based, community oriented and has a preventative focus).

From primary medical care to public health organisation?

Within the Health Management Group at City University, we asked 'Masterclass' participants to undertake a brief exercise to explore their understanding of primary care, by completing the following statements:

- primary care was. . . . . . (in 1988)
- primary care is . . . . (in 1998)
- primary care will be . . . . (in 2008).

(Meads and Cornish 1998)

The outcome of this exercise was illuminating. Participants saw 1988 as a kind of 'golden age' for primary care (notwithstanding some of the challenges, for example, from the Cumberledge report on community nursing, and the GP contract implemented in response to *Promoting Better Health*). This period was viewed as one in which the GP sat at the top of a pyramid of professionals, and acted as the 'gatekeeper' to everything else – not only to secondary care, but also to other members of the primary care team.

The 'downside' of this was its perceived paternalism, and its (medical) professional domination.

Contemporary primary care was viewed as more of a 'hotch potch' – with fundholding and non-fundholding practices, single-handed and group practices, a myriad of 'pilot' schemes (TPPs, PCPs etc.). The focus was felt to have shifted towards more team working, though this was also perceived as variable, and, even within the primary care team, the GP was still in charge! This period was experienced by participants as a period of confusion, with a sense of being in the middle of a profound change. This perception was certainly right, as in the two years since the seminar, whilst many of the PCAP pilots have continued, GP fundholding has been abolished, PCGs established and PCTs introduced.

When asked to imagine the future for primary care, 'Masterclass' participants foresaw radical transformation. A much more team-based approach, both within and beyond the primary care organisation was envisaged. 'Primary care will be a public health organisation, rooted in the local community, and locked into the wider health agenda', remarked one participant. 'An "upside-down" organisation, with the primary care team supported by the GP' was another vision.

This vision contrasts sharply with recent research into the development of a public health model of primary care, in which the authors observe:

> In primary care, the traditional organisational basis of the GP practice centred around the independent contractor's status of the GP, is based on a small business model and individualistic approach. This does not promote collaborative working between practice professionals and other agencies. (Taylor *et al.* 1998: p. 62).

Will the transition to PCGs and PCTs overcome this? If so, how? What will need to change?

A partnership of opposites?

Public health and primary care do not, at first glance, seem to have much in common. Indeed, the history of both professional groups reveals some old rivalries and 'turf wars' – for example, during the first half of the twentieth century, when Medical Officers of Health located in the local authorities took on responsibility for maternal and child health, GPs 'complained bitterly of "encroachment" by public health doctors into what they saw as their domain, the treatment of individual patients'. (Lewis, in Holland *et al.* 1991.)

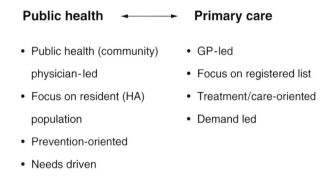

Public health ◄————► **Primary care**

- Public health (community)
  physician-led
- Focus on resident (HA)
  population
- Prevention-oriented
- Needs driven

- GP-led
- Focus on registered list
- Treatment/care-oriented
- Demand led

Figure 5.3 Public health and primary care perspectives.

More recently, the different tasks and perspectives of public health and primary care have frequently been conceptualised by as being at opposite ends of a spectrum, as illustrated in Figure 5.3.

However, closer analysis suggests that this conceptualisation of the difference between public health and primary care has some major flaws. First, it assumes that both public health and primary care are unitary concepts, with clear boundaries, that remain constant over time and place. As we have seen from the brief overview of the history of both, this is not the case. Public health and primary care have contested definitions – with ideas about what they are, what they do, and even who should do it, changing over time. The presentation of both as being at the opposite ends of the population/individual focus are, it could be argued, rooted in attempts by both public health physicians and general practitioners to 'carve out' their particular professional domains in relation to local communities, and in opposition to secondary (hospital-based) care.

As such, the different tasks and perspectives outlined above, fail to reflect the complexity of the work of either public health or primary care teams, both of which are (and to some extent have always been) multi-professional and inter-disciplinary in approach.

Furthermore, even limiting this conceptualisation to a representation of the two 'leading' players, that is, public health medicine and general practice (*see*, for example, Harris and Marshall 1997: pp. 10–11), there is still evidence of stereotyping. This was evident in the research undertaken by the HMG and Relationships Foundation for *Mixing Oil and Water* (Meads *et al.* 1999), where we found primary care participants who were well versed in public health issues, who took a population focus and who were already developing partnerships for health with their local communities.

The current cultures of primary care and public health may indeed appear to be very different, but there is nothing fixed about this difference –

change is possible, inevitable and already in process. Furthermore, a closer look reveals a range of similarities. These organisations contain within them a range of subcultures – for example, many primary care teams include community nurses and health visitors who are trained in public health, just as many public health departments have public health nurses who have worked in the community, and even public health doctors who have undergone GP training. In many cases, there may be as many similarities as differences, and it is to some of these similarities that we will turn next. For PCTs, understanding the subcultural subtext is all-important.

The task ahead

Public health professionals are currently just as caught up in organisational change as their colleagues in primary care. The roles and responsibilities of public health departments are undergoing reassessment in response to the ambitious health improvement agenda set out in *Saving Lives*. Public health teams are being required to work in partnership with local government and the wider local community, as well as being responsible for meeting the public health needs of primary care. At the same time, they also have to ensure that essential ongoing work is maintained. Many departments are in the throes of debate around the tension between having a 'critical mass' of public health skills in one place, versus the need to be sensitive to local communities, or reconfiguring around the new PCTs. It is hardly surprising, therefore, that many public health departments are feeling that their current capacity is being considerably stretched, and that some are feeling the need to learn new skills and new ways of working (Meads *et al.* 1999).

But the emphasis of the new public health agenda is that it is a 'joined-up' policy agenda at all levels. Neither public health nor primary care is being expected to deliver alone. There are enormous opportunities for sharing skills and expertise, and for transferable learning, between and within organisations. The public health 'system' is larger than either NHS public health or primary care (Table 5.1).

At the time of writing, health authorities retain overall responsibility for public health. Directors of Public Health are expected to continue providing strategic leadership and advocacy on public health issues, but PCG/Ts will be expected to make use of a wide range of specialist public health skills to support them in the following tasks:

- assessing the need for healthcare in their local communities
- contributing to the development and implementation of the HImP

Table 5.1 The public health system

Wider public health	Public healthcare	Public health specialist
Regional offices • Performance management • Finance directors • R&D managers • Plus managers and administrative staff in other RO directorates	• Primary care development team • Strategic/corporate development • Education and training leads • Postgraduate deans • Organisation & development leads • CHC co-ordinators	• Public health doctors & trainees • Public health specialists (other disciplines) • Dental public health • OHN co-ordinator • Public health nursing • Pharmaceutical advisers • Information specialists
Health authorities • Finance Director • IT and information staff • Child protection officer • Human resource staff (including training co-ordinators) • Communication staff • Other key administrative staff	• Primary care development staff • Strategic/corporate development • Health authority representatives on education and training consortia • Drugs action teams • HIV co-ordinators • Audit staffu (inc. MAAG)	• Public health doctors & trainees • Public health specialists (other disciplines) • Dental public health & trainees • Health promotion specialists • Public health nurses • Pharmaceutical advisers • Information specialists • Epidemiologists • Health economists • Social scientists • Research assistants • OHN/HImP co-ordinators
Primary care • Chief Officers • Training co-ordinators • Primary care development • Facilitators/managers	• GPs • Heath visitors/midwives • Community/practice nurses • PAMs	• Clinical governance leads • Health promotion specialists • 'Attached' public health staff
NHS trusts • Chief Executive • Trust board (executive) • Non-executive members	• Medical director • Clinical staff • Health visitors • Community nurses	• Health promotion specialists • Community dentists/dental public health • Infection control nurses • TB nurses • CCS (laboratory staff)

Continued

Table 5.1 Continued

Wider public health	Public healthcare	Public health specialist
Local authorities • Chief executives • Directors of all local authority departments • Teachers & other school staff • Care managers	• School nurses • Education psychologist • Education welfare officers • Youth service • Personal and sexual education advisers/teachers • Social workers • Environmental health officers • Housing department staff • Transport • Leisure services	• Environmental health • Health promotion • Health policy officers
Academic departments • Staff delivering courses such as NVQs & GNVQs in health and healthcare, and other professional training programmes – e.g. for nurses, health visitors & professions allied to medicine		• CsPHM/honorary lecturers • Lecturers in other core disciplines (epidemiology, statistics, health economics, sociology of health and illness, sociology of medicine, health psychology, health policy, health promotion)

Source: Cornish and Russell 1998.

- ensuring that services are based on evidence of clinical and cost-effectiveness
- inter-agency work on public health issues
- health promotion, screening and health protection
- community development.

As PCTs continue to develop, a range of public health roles and responsibilities may be devolved to them, although arrangements for public health surveillance (including the prevention and control of communicable diseases, and the maintenance of cancer registries) will not be delegated for the foreseeable future.

So, all primary care organisations will need to develop a range of public health skills and competencies to support them in their work in a number of areas, including:

- promoting health
- preventing disease
- assessing local health needs
- evaluating local health services
- encouraging evidence-based policy making
- supporting evidence-based clinical practice
- implementing clinical governance
- prioritising services
- setting health improvement targets
- monitoring progress towards those targets.

Building capacity to deliver health improvement

But what will this mean in practice? What are 'public health skills and competencies'? Who has them now, and how can primary care develop them? This has, inevitably, been the subject of much discussion, within and beyond to public health profession. A number of national and regional projects have looked at developing public health capacity and capability, and the skills and competencies needed to deliver the new agenda.

Box 5.4   Public health competency framework

- Surveillance and assessment of the health of the population
- Protecting and promoting health and wellbeing, including communicable disease control and environmental health
- Managing knowledge and getting research evidence into practice
- Managing, analysing and interpreting information and statistics
- Professional advice
- Developing and influencing policy
- Communicating with the public: public health advocacy
- Strategic leadership for health across all sectors
- Working with all sectors which impact on health and healthcare
- Prioritising in health and healthcare
- Developing quality and an evaluative culture
- Education and research

Source: Faculty of Public Health Medicine 2000

Workforce development for public health is high on the agenda of the Department of Health, the Faculty of Public Health Medicine, the Health Development Agency and other professional groups. The competency framework (Box 5.4) developed by the Faculty of Public Health Medicine, although designed for public health medicine trainees, summarises some of the key competencies required for public health practice and is a valuable tool for PCTs to use in their local community development programmes.

Primary care trusts: the options/opportunities for everyone

The public health challenge is not confined to either public health or to primary care. Delivering *Saving Lives: our healthier nation* will have an impact on the public health resources available at all levels, and many of the current tensions between different professional groups and different organisational cultures may well become more exaggerated before their creative potential can be released. Nevertheless, many of the roles and responsibilities which PCG/Ts are being expected to take on are not entirely new – public health and health promotion staff elsewhere within (and in many cases, beyond) the NHS have already developed skills and competencies in these areas. The issue is how these skills and competencies can be best deployed in new organisations, and it is here that the issue of transferable learning is most useful.

References

Acheson D (Chair) (1988) *Public Health in England: report of the Committee of Enquiry into the future development of the public health function.* HMSO, London.

Ashton J and Seymour H (1988) *The New Public Health.* Open University Press, Milton Keynes.

Black C (1999) Public health and health promotion. In: S Griffiths and D Hunter (eds) *Perspectives in Public Health.* Radcliffe Medical Press, Oxford.

Cornish Y (2001) *Public health and health promotion* (PhD thesis). City University. Unpublished.

Cornish Y and Griffiths F (1993) *Public Health and Primary Care: report to the Regional Directors of Public Health Group.* South West Thames RHA, London.

Cornish Y and Russell C et al. (1997) *Review of Health of the Nation in North Thames.* South East Institute of Public Health, Tunbridge Wells.

Cornish Y and Russell C (1998) *Implementing Health Strategy – some key issues underlying multi-agency approaches.* Proceedings of the Faculty of Public Health Medicine Annual Scientific Meeting, Torquay.

Department of Health (1988) *Health of the Population: responsibilities of health authorities* (HC(88)64). Department of Health, London.

Department of Health (1990) *Working for Patients* (Cm 555). HMSO, London.

Department of Health (1992) *The Health of the Nation: a strategy for England.* HMSO, London.

Department of Health and Social Security (1987) *Promoting Better Health: the Government's programme for improving primary health care* (Cm 249). HSMO, London.

Dubos R (1984) The mirage of health. In: N Black, D Boswell, A Gray *et al.* (eds) *Health and Disease.* Open University Press, Milton Keynes.

Faculty of Public Health Medicine (2000) *Standards for Public Health Physicians.* Consultation paper from the working group on record of in-service training assessment. FPHM, London.

Harris A and Marshall T (1997) The language of needs assessment. In: A Harris (ed) *Needs to Know: a guide to needs assessment for primary care.* Churchill Livingstone, London.

Holland W, Detels R and Knox G (1991) *Oxford Textbook of Public Health.* Oxford University Press, Oxford.

Lalond M (1974) *A New Perspective on the Health of Canadians.* Minister of Supply and Services, Ottowa.

Meads G and Cornish Y (1998) *Aids for Developing Primary Care Organisations* (Workbook for the Capita Masterclass). Health Management Group, City University, London.

Meads G, Killoran A, Ashcroft J and Cornish Y (1999) *Mixing Oil and Water.* Health Education Authority, London.

Moon G and North N (2000) *Policy and Place – general medical practice in the UK.* Macmillan, Basingstoke.

NHS Executive (1998a) *Primary Care Groups: delivering the agenda.* Department of Health, Leeds.

NHS Executive (1998b) *Shared Contribution, Shared Benefits* (HSC 1998/116). Department of Health, Leeds.

NHS Executive (1999) *Primary Care Trusts: establishment, the preparatory period and their functions.* Department of Health, Leeds.

Secretary of State for Health (1999) *Saving Lives: our healthier nation* (Cm 4386). HMSO, London.

Taylor P, Peckham S and Turton P (1998) *A Public Health Model of Primary Care – from concept to reality.* Public Health Alliance, Birmingham.

Tudor Hart J (1984) A new kind of doctor. In: N Black, D Boswell, A Gray *et al.* (eds) *Health and Disease.* Open University Press, Milton Keynes.

World Health Organization (1978) *Report of the International Conference on Primary Health Care, Alma Ata 1977.* WHO, Geneva.

World Health Organization (1985) *Targets for Health for All.* WHO, Copenhagen.

CHAPTER 6

Getting to grips with
social services

Rosie Benaim

The old divisions between health and social care need to be overcome.[1]

Introduction

The material presented in this chapter illuminates the current role of social services departments, and local authorities in general, in PCGs and their potential contribution to emerging NHS PCTs. It looks at how well-equipped social services departments are to participate; highlights obstacles; considers the potential within social services for helping to develop local health agendas; and clarifies some of the conditions that are necessary in order for local authorities to fully operate as equal partners in the task of planning an integrated healthcare service for their populations.

As well as examples from local authorities, the chapter refers to the history of social care–health services collaboration: the professional and organisational factors that have affected how this has developed previously; and what cultural 'baggage' both partners bring to this new venture in primary care service development.

Context

This chapter draws on material from a study of how two local anonymised English authorities, 'Southborough' and 'Northchester', approached their involvement in the setting up of PCGs. It examines that process, mindful of the context in which these emerging primary care organisations operate; that is, a context in which multi-disciplinary primary care organisations are charged with the responsibility for assessing the needs of local

---

[1] *NHS Plan* 2000: 7.1

populations and planning and commissioning their health services. These organisations have arisen in an environment in which primary care has gained prominence within the NHS, where a move away from the medical model of health to a more social model has led to a greater acceptance among healthcare professionals of a holistic idea of 'health', and where the stage is now set for closer collaboration between health and social care.

The development of community care in the last 20 years has led to an increased acceptance among health and social care workers of the practical necessity for closer collaboration, as they work increasingly closely together in the field maintaining vulnerable, often multiply disabled people in the community, living 'ordinary lives'.

The new Labour government has vigorously now urged all public sector organisations to work together to reduce the forces that produce 'social exclusion' – such as poverty, ill-health and poor education. The modernisation agenda within both the NHS and local government aims to ensure that organisations in the field of health and welfare work together, drop artificial barriers and co-operate in the planning and provision of services which promote health and reduce inequalities. The principle overarching this new 'partnership working' is that public services should be locally relevant and locally accountable. *Our Healthier Nation* (Department of Health 1998a), *Saving Lives* (Department of Health 1999) and *Partnership in Action* (Department of Health 1998b) all urge closer health–social care collaboration so that flexible arrangements can facilitate healthy communities. Such other government papers as, for example, *Modernising Health and Social Services: national priorities guidance 1999–00/2001–02* (Department of Health 1998c) urge not just closer working but a bringing together of health and social care as one force, and the *NHS Plan 2000* paves the way for fully-fledged Care Trusts in the mid-term. The Parliamentary Health Select Committee's report *The Relationship between Health and Social Services* (Health Select Committee Report 1998) vigorously argued for the complete integration of the two services, although it noted that, 'the involvement of social services departments and community NHS trusts in PCGs and PCTs provides an excellent opportunity for improved collaboration between health and social services, but falls well short of unifying the two agencies'.

Entering PCGs – social services' story

There is a long history attached to aligning social and health services. Prior to the reforms emanating from the 1968 Seebohm Committee (HMSO 1968) certain social work services were based within the health sector. With the subsequent social services departments lodging within the democratically accountable system of the local authority, and the development of generic social work a divide developed both at an operational and structural level. Over the last 30 years, moves have taken place to bridge the gap. Northern Ireland has integrated health and social services departments and in some fields, notably learning difficulties and mental health services, health and social services have seen the practical benefits of closer working, even of joint funding and joint management of services. The Health Act 1999 allows pooling of health and local authority budgets for the provision of combined health and social care services and this opens up opportunities for fully integrated services staffed and managed by the NHS and social services departments jointly.

It is therefore nothing new for social services departments to be asked to participate in a joint venture with the health service. But the new PCG/T set up differs considerably from any of the previous models as it has a far wider remit and requires broader partnership working than anything previously conceived. It is not just about developing easier operational relations, it is about forming a large multi-agency organisation which plans and commissions local health services.

PCG boards consist of GP representatives (up to seven), community nursing representatives (up to two), one LA representative (almost invariably from the social services department) and a lay representative. As the boards were being established in 1998, local authorities were required to nominate a board representative for each PCG within their authority. *Good Practice Guidelines* published belatedly by the Association of Directors of Social Services in June 1999 referred to the social services department representative having 'particular responsibility in relation to social care matters, [though] their involvement should also facilitate consideration of wider local authority issues such as the social, economic and environmental links with health improvement and action to tackle health inequality'.

'Southborough' Local Authority

Southborough's profile

- Outer London borough covering a range of poorer, inner-city type communities and more affluent suburban areas.
- Labour-controlled council.
- Three PCGs – all operating at level 2.
- Three SSD PCG representatives, all 'third tier' managers, *viz.* disabilities services manager, hospital and health liaison services manager and home care services manager. (Assistant director for adult services deputised for a time as PCG representative, as one representative retired.)

Documentation relating to Southborough Social Services Department's involvement in PCGs

The local authority's own guidelines for PCG representation emphasised the need for the board member to represent the local authority, not just the social services department. It stipulated that representatives should be involved in local needs assessment and the development of service and commissioning strategies; advising on social services and local authority matters and promoting a whole systems approach to health and social care. The guidelines allowed the social services role on PCG boards to develop along a range from informing and advising through to planning and commissioning, so permitting the social services representatives to take on a wide range of duties and a broad spectrum of responsibility, from acting as an advocate for social services users to designing services and commissioning resources.

In a paper referring to the HImP (Health Improvement Programme), the Assistant Director of Social Services referred to the need for PCG board members to keep abreast of HImP developments in view of its ability to reflect a single coherent plan, the effectiveness of pooling budgets and new initiatives, along with the ability of agencies to deliver less 'boundaried' and more efficient services to the community. It also pointed to the HImP's capacity to act as a focus for better NHS and social service collaboration in the co-ordination and integration of services for priority groups.

A consultation document on establishing PCGs by the health authority quotes NHS Executive guidance on the aim of building better health alliances between GPs and the wider health community. This included local government, recognising the inclusion of social services on PCG governing bodies as important in relation to putting in place, and possibly providing, integrated care packages for individuals and co-ordinating health and social services locally. A PCG implementation group included local authority representation alongside health authority, NHS trust, GP and community health council representatives. The local authority representative on that body liaised with the local authority representatives on the HImP co-ordinating group (which has responsibility for drawing up the Health Action Zone bid), and on the 'Health Assembly' standing conference, which is concerned with the planning and implementation of the HImP and joint planning issues involved in it.

At the end of 1998, a one-day conference facilitated by a London university was held involving all PCG board members and other interested partners in the health and local authorities and voluntary sector. Workshops at the conference allowed board members to air issues of concern and share ideas.

The perspective of Southborough Local Authority's SSD on their involvement in PCGs

One PCG representative reported in mid-1998 that she felt the PCG agenda was very medically focused, and was concerned with matters such as the transfer of secondary care services to primary care and how GP board members were funded and designated. Having had considerable experience of work with the local total purchasing project (TPP), she felt that at that point the PCG was like 'the TPP rewritten'. In those early days she found it hard to imagine how the PCT board would be formed and at what level it would operate.

The view of the Assistant Director of Social Services was that a well established tradition of close health and social services co-working in the authority had provided a sound basis for the establishment of PCGs. For example, close working between community nurses and the home care service is in place. She felt that the PCG board allowed the SSD representatives to share their skills with other board members and that joint planning happens easily at board level. Before more ambitious aims of joint commissioning and budget pooling can be approached, however, she felt working relations must be properly established. Her view was that SSD representatives use the boards to inform the NHS about local authority activities which affect or ally to PHC work. She felt that the local authority had taken considerable care to ensure that the three representatives feel well informed and supported in their role as board members. A PCG project board of senior officers provides this support to the board members. This includes the Assistant Director for Children's Services, a planning unit officer who advises on community care, children's services and joint commissioning, and a finance officer who provides information on financial and purchasing issues.

A third representative reported towards the end of 1999 that the PCG agenda was very fixed on clinical governance and, still, on the mechanics of setting up the board. The primary care investment plan, prescribing budgets and general structures were more important than SSD collaboration. While feeling he was of equal status to the other board representatives, he pointed out that he was only one while there are seven GPs. His view was that the health members on the board can sometimes see social services' relevance to the board's work as obscure. For example, one GP queried why a local Surestart co-ordinator had made a presentation to the board, as the business of Surestart is not specifically medical. (Surestart is a national initiative to address the health and developmental needs of pre-school children.) Generally, he felt that social services' work is seen as allied, but separate to the work of the PCG. A team-building day for the board, in his view, let members get acquainted with each other and begin to understand the different agencies' responsibilities and perspectives. The PCG work he undertakes is regarded as an 'add on' to his other work and can be a pressure given his normal management and service delivery duties. Needing to be acquainted with the broad range of issues is a further pressure. As well as being a board member, he is also a member of several of the board's subgroups. He summed up by expressing the view that the PCG set up was still evolving; that social services is taking a 'wait and see' line; and that while being engaged in the process, he is still not sure what the final structure, nor what social services' expected role within it will be.

'Northchester' Local Authority
Northchester's profile

- Metropolitan district council in the north of England with a mix of inner city, urban and rural communities.
- Labour-controlled council.
- Four PCGs at level 2.
- Four social services PCG representatives, of which three are third tier managers (area managers for elderly services) and one a second tier manager, the Assistant Director for Older People.

Documentation relating to Northchester District Council's involvement in PCGs

The Director of Social Services in a conference address in 1998 drew attention to the local authority role on PCG boards and in PCGs as planning and commissioning bodies. He pointed to a number of issues and areas of concern. These were:

- health and social service collaboration within a medically-oriented organisation
- acknowledging the vast resources – financial, material and staff – that a local authority will bring to a PCG
- the democratic deficit in PCGs and how this may conflict with local authority traditions.

Prior to the PCGs running in full form from April 1999, the health authority organised a number of workshops to assist PCG board members assimilate their new range of responsibilities. Two of 14 workshops were specifically aimed at involving the social services representative. The first aimed to develop awareness among GPs, social services, non-executive directors and lay people of the role and function of a PCG and each other's roles. The second focused particularly on the role of the social services representative and addressed the skills the social services representative would need to perform in the PCG set up.

In a reply to the health authority's initial proposals for PCGs configuration, the Director of Social Services replied by pointing out how reconfiguring social services' team boundaries in line with PCG boundaries might destroy patch-based social services teams. It welcomed the development of PCGs as vehicles to provide improved health services for local people and also made reference to the potential situation of elected members of PCT boards which would be legally independent from the health authority.

The district's HAZ bid sought to prove that a 'joined-up' approach also existed to addressing poor health and health inequalities by describing a complex but robust framework through which the health and local authorities, NHS trusts, voluntary sector, local university and community health councils would address health priorities and institute systems which allow curative, preventive and health promotion measures to be implemented. Health and social services collaboration was presented as commonplace in service provision and the new PCG system welcomed as a way in which HAZ initiatives could be promoted on the ground.

An 'action plan' for the district's inner-city PCG, written by the social services department's PCG representative, outlined the board's objectives and aspirations. Nine key tasks were stipulated including the development of primary care, reducing accidents and developing clinical governance arrangements. In only one key task – the development of mental health services – was the PCG working with social services specifically given special mention. Partnership working in the other key tasks referred to 'local government partners' and the local authority being one of the local organisations that the PCG should 'identify, develop, nurture and maintain collaborative relationships, agreements and understandings with'.

The perspective of Northchester's SSD reps on their PCG involvement

The Director of Social Services in mid-1998 anticipated benefits and difficulties in the establishment of PCGs. The district has a long and well established history of health and social care joint working initiatives. The character of the PCGs in the district, it was anticipated, would vary, e.g. from poor inner city with many single-handed GPs to other areas where disparate communities would present problems for the principle of configuring PCGs on a 'natural community' basis. He looked to the development of HAZ initiatives to take forward any plans for closer health and social care relations and as the vehicle to address the issue of 'healthy communities'. The Director saw the need for senior and experienced SSD officers as the PCG board representatives so that PCG boards could be well-informed about local authority services in general. He saw their role also as promoting within the developing PCG structure the social care culture of 'individuals mattering' and 'ordinary life' principles. He felt that senior social services managers have the ability to, and must become *au fait* with the language, terms and mindset of health planners so that they can comprehensively represent social services and the local authority in general in this new forum.

The PCG manager for people with disabilities was specifically concerned about how PCG structures would affect the planning and commissioning of services for specialist groups, e.g. younger people with disabilities, fearing they might cause inequity of provision from one PCG to another. North-chester Social Services Department at present has specific service planning mechanisms to ensure user groups' specialist needs are met and he is keen these are not lost.

The Assistant Director for Disability and Community Health was concerned that PCG boards understand, and are linked into, the current range of joint planning and joint commissioning structures. The HAZ locally has come to operate as a controlling initiative, moulding other services and determining the overall direction of health and social services' joint work. PCGs are encouraged to develop their own 'mini-HAZs'. Similarly, local HImPs will attempt to integrate their own specific local needs with borough-wide plans. Accordingly, the PCG boards can expect to have to find their level in a pattern of inter-agency joint planning bodies whose agendas may coincide or conflict. She believes local authority PCG board representatives bring management, budget-holding, and community planning expertise to the boards, and their knowledge of local voluntary and private sector services is unique among board members. A post to support the SSD representatives on PCG/Ts funded by the HAZ is proposed.

The Assistant Director for Older People (member of the inner-city PCG board) felt his most important job was educating other board members about local authority services, through sharing expertise in making local needs assessments, networking with community partners and consulting with user groups. Local authority knowledge of 'quality' issues helps PCGs in their clinical governance discussions. Building on essentially good health and social services relations, he felt that social services had been 'first to the table' by nominating its representatives before GPs and community nurses. His approach was to offer vigorous support and advice to the board in its early formative stages, advising on agenda setting and on operating as a board. Management skills, he felt, are what distinguish social services PCG board members from other board representatives, and contributing these skills to the process of establishing boards is important in helping establish SSD credibility on the boards. On his board he leads on commissioning and produced the board's Vision Statement.

The health authority Assistant Director's perspective on social services' involvement in PCGs acknowledged that boards see social services' involvement as useful and that the links with the community, the expertise in resource and staff management, planning, and commissioning skills provided by social services representatives are all highly valued. She questioned, however, whether or not grassroots workers in primary medical care, hospital and community trusts and the local authority itself understood the how and why of social services' involvement in PCGs. The different level of development of each PCG affects the way in which the social services representative is viewed and utilised on the board. One board is very clinically driven in its service development focus, and has not got beyond that issue. Another is focusing on establishing itself as an organisation that can communicate in the health setting, whereas another PCG accepts a much broader definition of 'health' and is able to look to making wider links with local authority and other community organisations. With regard to the effect of the HAZ on the development of PCG services, she felt that the HAZ agenda in the district has become quite bureaucratic and planning focused. She feels that any differences it has made on the ground are not yet evident, so on this basis she could not comment on how the HAZ initiatives are impacting upon service planning within PCGs. While the considerable skills SSD managers have in management, planning and commissioning are seen to be a real benefit to PCGs, she would not want PCGs to become too bureaucratic and hide-bound by procedures, protocols and regulations.

Summary

The material gathered from 'Southborough' and 'Northchester' shows overall a positive and energetic input from the social services departments into the establishment of local PCGs. Officers of considerable seniority are putting time and energy into their role as board members, often serving on board subgroups and taking on specific planning roles for the PCG. In both local authorities, however, the overall sense was of the social services PCG representatives being slightly removed from the main business of the board in its present form – for example, prescribing budgets and supporting GP locum arrangements figured more in board discussions than ways of jointly commissioning health and social care services. Health professional PCG board members may see social services as an important support for local health services, but still do not necessarily see health and social care as being in the 'health business' to the same degree.

Collaborative working between health and social services is seen as vital operationally, but joint planning and commissioning of health services by health and social services is still not readily widely understood or accepted. The SSDs appear to find that 'standing on the sidelines' is acceptable at the moment, feeling that the establishment of working PCG/T boards is primarily an NHS task in which they can offer support and assistance, but from which they stand slightly apart.

Key elements in social service involvement in PCG/Ts

- The majority of health sector representatives may not see social services as being in 'the health business', nor appreciate social services' potential contribution to developing health services for localities.
- This health sector may consider that social service involvement in PCG/Ts is in order to progress collaborative *operational* work, not to join in joint commissioning.
- Tensions in working relationships between health and social services staff which arise in the field may transfer to interactions on the board.
- Individual social services representatives may find their PCG/T board work burdensome alongside their other departmental duties if the two fail to coalesce.
- One social services representative on a board may feel swamped by the large number of health sector representatives.
- Health sector representatives may perceive social services departments as very bureaucratic in their accountabilities and administration and resist these characteristics transferring to the PCG/T structures.
- Social services are contributing to setting up new primary care organisations, but feel they are playing a waiting game and their role will not become clear for some time.
- Explicit discussions at board level are helpful about SSD representatives' functions and potential on the board.
- The PCG/T agendas are often currently still about medical services with the health sector in the driving seat.

- As multi-million pound, multi-agency organisations, local authorities potentially have a central role in the planning and commissioning of local health services – while understood at a senior strategic level, this may not be fully appreciated among board members yet.
- The local authority, with and through its social services department, should explicitly acknowledge how it perceives its role and function within PCG/Ts.
- Board chief executives and chairs need to encourage and promote social services participation in order to fully exploit its potential in local health service planning and commissioning.

PCT's capacity to develop and promote health and social care co-working

Establishing PCGs over a two-year period has given SSDs a chance to rehearse their role within these new primary care organisations. While central government may urge public services to work together to develop locally relevant health services, the practical realities of how boards organise to plan, commission and fund services will in the end determine what level of responsibility and influence the local authority has within primary care planning and development through PCTs.

Health and social services antipathy may carry over to board activities (for example professional and organisational differences can cause tensions). Research by Khan *et al.* (1998) showed that GPs can see no active role for social services in PCG/Ts in strategic planning and commissioning although the value of collaboration is acknowledged at an operational level. GP/SSD co-operation at board level may be affected if this is the case, especially if, as Rummery (1998) discovered, there is within PCTs no incentive for the NHS to collaborate in commissioning with social services. The King's Fund Joint Commissioning Project (1999) warned that, often in health and social services joint commissioning, little attention is paid to the 'specific outcomes' that the different partners wish to achieve by working together and the process of working together is seen as an end in itself. Health and social services co-working on PCTs must not become just another example of working together being seen as an end in itself.

As PCGs evolve into PCTs and social services representatives continue to have a central position on the new Executive Committees, it is important for boards to examine the potential of the local authority within the PCT structure. Social services departments are in the business of health in its broadest sense and if PCTs wish to meet the needs of their localities, then it is important to harness the knowledge, skills and resources of the local authority in that task.

Working models – a checklist for social services' involvement in primary care organisations

The following three models, with attached action plans, show how social services' involvement in PCTs might be approached and may help boards consider where social services' involvement in the PCT currently and potentially lies. It is based on a wide range of individual contemporary case examples, including those detailed earlier in this chapter.

Model 1 – Antagonistic model

In this model negative elements in health and social services' relations dominate (e.g. different professional judgements, separated organisational arrangements), and health and social service parties are unable to agree common purpose. The health service does not see a role for social services in healthcare provision and both parties see each other as rivals not partners in the enterprise.

Action plan for Model 1

- Institute systems and working groups to establish good, basic working relations, and promote familiarity and understanding of each other's roles, powers and structures.
- Reframe professional contributions and tensions as positive individual contributions to a diverse collective direction.
- Ensure that the board as a whole addresses the role of the local authority in the PCG/T, so that the local authority perspective, resources and skills are incorporated into every aspect of the group/trust's work.

Model 2 – Doctor–handmaiden model

The social services department views its role as one of supporting the NHS. SSDs and local authorities generally see themselves as peripheral to the task of providing health services and consider their role as the giving of support and co-operation to the health service in its task of providing core medical services. Social services try to be as accommodating as possible in collaborative work and provide a supportive social care element to certain health services, e.g. elderly and mental health services. Social services' involvement is in playing a supporting role to the main act – the NHS and health.

Action plan for Model 2

- Guard against complacency by ensuring that the social services/local authority is involved in all possible areas of the PCG/T's work.
- Social services representatives must resist any pressure to have their role and function defined by the health and medical services in the PCG/T and ensure their unique contribution is not distorted or lost.
- Focus on the local authority capacity to be involved in joint commissioning; do not be satisfied only with achieving good operational joint working.
- There should be general acceptance that the SSD's role is at the heart of decision-making, not restricted to supportive and advisory functions.

Model 3 – Equal partners model

In this, all the NHS representatives and the local authority together reassess what is 'health' and view the achievement of a healthy community as one in which medical services, social services, education, housing and environmental health along with a multitude of other statutory and voluntary organisations all have valuable and equally important roles to play. The venture into developing PCTs and future Care Trusts is then one of real partnership in which all views are equally valued and the task is seen as that of developing a network of interrelated services which complement and enhance each other. This is not a model in which one service is the core and centre with others as its satellites, but one in which each service is both interdependent and complementary.

Action plan for Model 3

- Ensure all systems involve multi-disciplinary and multi-professional consultation and planning and allow local authority councillors, users and carers to participate in planning and commissioning structures.
- Invest in maintaining the robust structures required and ensure personnel have the time and opportunity to maintain easy communication, consultation and joint working.

Conclusion

There is no doubt that the local authority presence on PCG boards and within the new PCT structures is both essential and valued. There is a danger, however, that because of the way PCGs developed in their first two or three years the role of SSDs and the local authority generally has not been fully examined within the PCG/T structure. For PCTs to progress and achieve their potential as multi-agency primary care organisations planning health services for local communities, the role of the local authority needs to be clarified and its skills and resources properly harnessed.

Like most models, the three cited in the previous section are caricatures. One is unlikely to come across real examples of health and social care working quite as crudely polarised as the antagonistic and the doctor–handmaiden models. Nor is the naive, uncompetitive, pure partnership of the equal partners model likely to see the light of day in contemporary local politics. Nevertheless, these models contain elements of the forces and influences at work in the current formation of PCTs and can serve as a checklist for boards to enable them to maximise local authority involvement and influence. If the first two models can try to work towards something more like the third model then government rhetoric on achieving healthy communities might stand a better chance of becoming a reality.

References

Department of Health (1998a) *Our Healthier Nation: a contract for health* (Cm 3852). HMSO, London.

Department of Health (1998b) *Partnership in Action: a discussion document.* HMSO, London.

Department of Health (1998c) *Modernising Health and Social Services: national priorities guidance 1999–00/2001–02.* HMSO, London.

Department of Health (1999) *Saving Lives: our healthier nation* (Cm 4386). HMSO, London.

Health Select Committee Report (1998) *The Relationship between Health and Social Services.* HMSO, London.

HMSO (1968) *Report of the Committee on Local Authority and Allied Personal Social Services* (Seebohm Report) (Cm 3703). HMSO, London.

Khan P, Lupton C, Lacey D *et al.* (1998) Primary care groups and partnerships with social services departments: the perspective of general practitioners. *Social Services Research*, The University of Birmingham. **3**: 19–28.

King's Fund (1999) *Partnerships between Health and Social Care.* Report of the King's Fund Joint Commissioning Project.

Rummery K (1998) Changes in primary health care policy: the implications for joint commissioning with social services. *Health Soc Care Community.* **6**(6): 429–37.

CHAPTER 7

Turning community hospitals into assets

Helen Tucker

A new range of intermediate care services will build a bridge between hospital and home.[1]

New primary care organisations, and in particular PCTs, have the opportunity to bring fresh thinking into the development, delivery and monitoring of local health services and in particular community hospitals. Taking the step from commissioning services to having a direct responsibility for the management of resources which include the staff, budget and even the estate of community hospitals, encourages a new approach to this service which is so highly valued by local people.

PCG/Ts are at varying levels of understanding and experience regarding community hospital services. A diversity of interests, experience, preferences and vision within a primary care organisation with regard to community hospital services is not uncommon. Primary care organisations (PCOs) looking for guidance on community hospitals will find a mixed picture. Drawing on our recent nationwide research, it is possible, however, to identify and draw on specific good practice that may be relevant to local circumstances.

National policy direction supports the development of health services 'closer to home', the third option described in *Shaping the Future NHS – long term planning for hospitals and related services* (Department of Health 2000). Criteria such as ease of access to services are recognised as crucial to the timely and appropriate use of services. *The New NHS: modern, dependable* made an explicit reference to community hospitals being used to the full in future, recognising that they had been sidelined in the past (Secretary of State 1997). The contribution that community hospital services can make to the management of the acute workload is becoming more widely acknowledged (Secretary of State 1997: p. 41; Jay *et al.* 1999; Vaughan and

---

[1] *NHS Plan* 2000: 1.18

Lathlean 1999; Secretary of State 2000). Community hospitals are considered to have a key role in intermediate care (Vaughan and Lathlean 1999) with services being based in or around the building and facilities. The service direction, ambitious targets and high investment levels for intermediate care as set out in the NHS Plan (Secretary of State 2000) give those concerned with promoting and developing the role of local hospitals a clear challenge.

Each community hospital service and population is unique, and national trends are not readily discernible. National strategies for these services have been absent in the past, and more recent locally produced strategies have had a mixed reception. Therefore, PCOs are taking their own individual approaches to the challenge to turn community hospitals into assets.

Alternative extended primary care service models and their viability

Community hospitals have often been viewed as an extension of the GP practice, offering the primary healthcare team an opportunity to extend the facilities they offered in their surgeries and health centres into such services as in-patient beds, out-patient clinics, diagnostic facilities, day services and minor injuries services. Definitions of community hospitals are inevitably being continually rewritten and updated, but a common feature in defining this model of service is that it benefits from the involvement of local medical staff (GPs) and serves a local, defined population (Department of Health 2000; Community Hospitals Association 1999). Four service models, as a result, have been categorised and labelled below as a guide. They are not mutually exclusive.

Community resource centre

This model describes the service as an integrated health and social care resource, with the hospital providing a focus for managing care which may be provided within the building, in a clinic, in a surgery or in the patient's home. The hospital as a community resource centre offers a base to community groups, voluntary agencies, self-help groups and complementary practitioners. It is typically a multi-provider facility, and may extend its scope to housing associations and local authorities. It is also a partnership model which is inclusive in design, very often with a high level of community involvement.

Primary resource centre

This model is an extension of the community resource centre, with GP primary care facilities within the centre. Typically this will be one or two practices or health centres at the hub of the resource centre, with the additional services as the spokes.

Intermediate care facility

This model concentrates on meeting the NHS intermediate care agenda, which is to provide a 'stage' or a 'level' of care between care in the surgery and care within a district general hospital (DGH). The patient categories for preventive intermediate care are set out in Box 7.1. Services will be designed to prevent unnecessary admissions to the DGH and to expedite discharge from the DGH. The services may be described as 'substitution', or 'complementary' to the work of the acute secondary care sector, and require a sophisticated interface between the services. Care pathways and shared care arrangements are examples of systems in use to support the process, so that GPs, consultant medical staff and nursing staff are working to an agreed plan in a managed way. The model encourages initiatives for step-up services (care for people currently living at home), and step-down services (care for patients being transferred from a secondary care hospital). Models of in-patient intermediate care include GP community beds, nurse-led community beds, nursing home beds with rehabilitation and social services transitional beds. Models of domiciliary intermediate care include intensive home support, confidence at home schemes, hospital at home schemes, rapid response teams, community rehabilitation teams and day services. These services are typically offered to patients who are medically stable and have a predicted episode of care. It is a service which may be

---

Box 7.1   Intermediate care

Community-based services designed to prevent medical dependence and promote personal independence
Types:
- prevention of A&E referrals (especially self-referrals)
- prevention of nursing/residential home admissions
- prevention of acute care hospital episodes
- prevention of hospital discharge delays.

Source: adapted from Steiner 1999

---

particularly appropriate for patients requiring general nursing care, palliative or terminal care and rehabilitative care, and fits the option of providing
'care closer to home' as described within the recent National Bed Inquiry
(Department of Health 2000).

Rehabilitation centre

A number of community hospitals stress their role in promoting independence, re-ablement and rehabilitation and health promotion and prevention
work. Many are proactive in working within their communities to support
healthy lifestyles through work with schools and colleges and in industry.

Models and viability

In practice, many community hospitals fulfil a variety of roles, and are
managed in such a way that local frameworks incorporate both integrated
intermediate care and community resource centre approaches. Testing for
viability for the models described above, or variations of these models,
requires a significant level of information on: local health and social care
needs; gaps and duplications in current services; a mapping of services for
access and availability; and financial resources. The process requires a sharing
of information between professionals, NHS providers and other local organisations. Examples of emerging models show that imagination and flair are also
key factors in considering service and financial viability. Those case studies
that are illustrated below have shared common themes of explicit values, a
clear understanding of appropriate care, a willingness to work in partnership, and flexibility and commitment to work with and for local people.

Potential NHS performance benefits and appropriate methods of option appraisal

Potential benefits

The NHS performance framework provides a common mechanism to work
to and provides a clear set of criteria against which existing and planned
services may be measured (NHS Executive 1999). Table 7.1 provides
examples of where this system has been applied. Providing evidence on
which to demonstrate the benefits requires a combination of hard data in

Table 7.1   National performance framework

Standards	Example
Health improvement	Multigym for older people established to help maintain and improve health, fitness and mobility (Leatherhead Hospital, Surrey)
Fair access to services	Extending catchment areas for GP beds with medical cover by nearby practice, so more local people can benefit (Newton-le-Willows Hospital, Liverpool)
Effective delivery of healthcare	Mobile gastroscopy unit set up to enable early diagnosis and treatment in an accessible way, with good use of staff resources and equipment (Honiton Hospital, Devon)
Efficiency	Nurse-led haematuria clinics to enable early diagnosis and intervention, with efficient use of medical and nursing time and limited visits by patients (Whitby Community Hospital, Yorkshire)
Patient and carer experience	Integrated health and social care day centre, with support for patients and carers (Patrick Stead Hospital, Suffolk)
Health outcomes of NHS care	Birthing unit evaluation showing lower levels of intervention and positive health outcomes for mothers and newborns in a midwife-led unit (Edgware Community Hospital, North London)

terms of statistics including activity and outcomes, as well as such soft data as satisfaction surveys. As in many areas of the NHS, there is much work to be done to provide a robust and proven case for future community hospital development. New PCTs are already putting pressure on the current systems by requiring reports in accordance with their new responsibilities and perspectives.

The Community Hospitals Association will be publishing the results of a survey (Community Hospitals Association and Department of Health, pending) funded by the Department of Health, that has identified examples of best practice and innovation in intermediate care in community hospitals. The examples in Table 7.1 are drawn from this study.

Option appraisal

A systematic approach to appraising options is becoming a requirement set by new primary care organisations, which are carrying out these exercises with local people, staff and other stakeholders as well as at management and policy levels. This inclusive approach makes the exercise more complex to manage, but the benefits of stakeholders owning, or taking a responsibility for the preferred option are very compelling.

The matrix in Table 7.2 is an example of an appraisal that was carried out for a primary care resource centre. The options and the criteria were established by an inter-agency steering group.

This simple option appraisal matrix has been adopted to help to address questions such as the following.

- Which organisation should manage the community hospital?
- Which services and facilities should be managed by the PCT?

Table 7.2 Example option appraisal with weightings for scores

Criteria	Weighting	Option 1	Option 2	Option 3	Option 4	Option 5
Is it acceptable to the community?	16					
Is it feasible?	14					
Does it offer quality of service?	14					
Does it offer value for money?	12					
Is it attractive to purchasers?	10					
Does it make best use of existing resources?	8					
Is it in keeping with national policy?	8					
Is it a long-term solution to health and care needs?	6					
Will it provide a satisfactory environment and safe clinical practice?	6					
Is it an accessible service?	6					
Total weighted score	**100**					

- Should the PCT manage the estates and facilities functions as well as clinical services?
- Which model of service best meets local need?

Key factors in successful development

The five factors normally shown to be significant, from our studies, in contributing to successful development are: community engagement; service design based on proven need; integration with social services; and a productive interface between NHS sectors and partnerships. Professor Joan Higgins, in her study on small hospitals in Britain (Higgins 1993), listed three key requirements for successful development, namely patient selection, appropriateness and the support of GPs. She has stressed that the service must have a defined role and work within appropriate boundaries according to known need. Professor Ritchie, in his study based in Scotland, also stresses the need to engage local people, have a clear strategy and development plan, and to ensure that there is strong GP support (Ritchie 1996).

Community engagement

This could fairly be described as the single most critical factor in progressing the development of community hospital services, and one which is appreciated by staff directly in contact with patients and carers including GPs, social services department staff, lay members and primary care practitioners on PCG/T boards. New primary care organisations are in many cases starting to address their responsibility for public accountability through such mechanisms as the engagement of local people in the planning of 'their' hospital.

Case study

Suffolk Health Authority undertook a collaborative exercise with local people when preparing a specification for a new provider for community hospitals. Over 100 people were actively involved in working groups to design a model for community hospitals. Local people took a lead in drawing on good practice, using research material, and visiting hospitals in the UK. The process was guided by clear principles, values and criteria. The emerging model was enthusiastically supported by local people, who wanted the selected provider to reconfigure the hospital services accordingly. The exercise was a valuable example of how to manage the complex process of engaging local people. It gave an appreciation of the need to support individuals who are not health professionals, provide information in a usable form, work to an explicit project plan and be clear about parameters and outcomes.

Service design based on proven need

Many PCG/Ts are instigating fresh reviews of health need, working in partnership with local authorities, voluntary and independent organisations and other commissioning, providing, campaigning and stakeholder organisations concerned with the health and regeneration of communities. Such studies are able to draw on a wide body of work, such as epidemiological analyses within public health agencies, local authority lifestyles studies, anti-poverty strategies, housing need studies by housing departments and housing associations, and other indices of need and social deprivation. Locally-based information can be used including GP practice profiles, caseloads of community and primary care staff and local audits, reviews and vulnerability indices. A fresh approach to collection, collation and interpretation of this information is starting to provide PCG/Ts with a basis for assessing priorities for investment and development, and also informing bids for additional resources, such as through single regeneration budget (SRB) applications from central government. As stated in the publication *Mixing Oil and Water*:

> The importance of new primary care organisations and public health initiatives aligning themselves together cannot be overstated. (Meads *et al.* 1999)

Many PCG/Ts are working proactively with a range of organisations and groups, enabling the Health Improvement Programme (HImP) to be influenced and shaped by local staff and local people interpreting and demonstrating local need.

Case study

West Barnet PCG instigated a health needs assessment for one practice as a pilot, prior to a rollout to all other practices. The area chosen has one of the highest levels of social deprivation in North London. The study incorporated all other work carried out by respective agencies, and brought this shared knowledge and learning into one document. From this, primary and community care staff validated the findings and enhanced the understanding of the community dynamics through case studies and examples. The result is an operational plan for the practice and the PCG, an understanding of how systems may be improved to provide more timely and appropriate information, and where priority investments may be made.

Integration with social services

This is a priority for NHS PCTs, and their Board constitutions encourage this. There are examples of community hospitals being turned from liabilities into assets following productive working with SSDs on a shared agenda. Particularly in remote areas, it may be that the population and health need is such that a specific hospital resource cannot be sustained. The community hospital is able to serve as a focus for health and social care as well as other associated functions and facilities. This is not to say that this model is a buildings-led model, but that the presence of an established focus for healthcare can be of benefit. Staff working within primary and community healthcare already have within their practice a working relationship with social services colleagues, and closer collaborations achieved through structures, policies, a shared environment, resources and other methods are being actively pursued.

Case study

When Rye Hospital, in East Sussex, was closed for financial and viability reasons against vigorous opposition, local people instigated a review which led to a feasibility and business case for a new service. The result was the Memorial Care Centre, which was a £5 million develop-ment led by the community in collaboration with health and social services, Shaftesbury Housing Association and voluntary groups. Aspects of integration with social services have included joint training, shared facilities, common assessments, multi-disciplinary, multi-agency reviews and flexible working across services provided by health and social services. Local people formed a charity to own and develop the centre, which has been running successfully for four years.

The productive interface between NHS sectors

This refers specifically to the interface between acute secondary care provided within the DGH, and primary and community care. The desired culture has changed dramatically from competition to collaboration, although in a number of instances this is still in theory rather than in practice. Community hospital developments can be encouraged through the acute sector's recognition of the value of the service, as often happens during periods of emergency pressures. The argument made in many quarters is that if a community hospital can enable the acute sector to concentrate on appropriate patients during periods of crisis, why can this way of working not be incorporated into general patterns? The development of jointly designed care pathways is helping to illustrate the benefits of planned and managed care, where patients may move swiftly through the acute sector, and have the appropriate rehabilitation, recovery and monitoring of care in a local facility.

Case study

Ulster Community & HSS Trust is a recently combined acute and community trust within the joint health and social care structure in Northern Ireland. A recent bed crisis in the acute sector prompted the emergency creation of a plan to accelerate patients through the acute sector into community and primary care settings. Within days, beds became available within the acute sector. None of the patients discharged was re-admitted to the acute sector. Improving patient flow through shared management of episodes is now being attended to as an integral part of the pattern of service.

Partnerships

Partnerships have been a very positive feature of community hospital developments, with examples of other organisations and agencies being involved in all aspects of planning, designing, developing, managing and monitoring community hospital services and facilities. One of the strongest partnerships is between the hospital and the community. Local people, through Leagues of Friends or similar charities, support their hospitals through fundraising, voluntary help, providing such services as libraries, coffee shops and transport, and by campaigning and bidding for resources and facilities. Examples of partnerships are hospice organisations who work with NHS staff to provide appropriate palliative and terminal care.

Case study

Dorothy House Hospice in Bradford-upon-Avon, Wiltshire, is a voluntary organisation with a team of skilled and specialist staff who support community staff in community hospitals in caring for people in their last illness. Dorothy House provides training courses, ongoing support and advice, and publications. The voluntary organisation has a very positive relationship with a number of NHS trusts in the area, and the results of joint working have been highly valued by staff and patients alike.

Common obstacles to successful development and how to address them

Five common obstacles experienced by new primary care organisations are: the lack of information; a historic shortage of investment in services and the environment; concern about clinical practice; the tensions around equity and access trade-offs; and the lack of financial and management resources. These obstacles are drawn from experience, recent surveys, and publications. In particular, Professor Lewis Ritchie's study of community hospitals in Scotland, and the Welsh Office study led by Dr Idris Humphrey set out these obstacles and others very clearly (Ritchie 1996; Humphrey *et al.* 1996).

Information

The lack of information is not peculiar to community hospital services, but is particularly marked because of the nature of the service. The service is usually considered to be an extension of primary care, and therefore recording at the hospital level can be viewed by medical staff as duplication of effort. The fact that so many are multi-provider sites means that the activity is managed by a range of organisations, with contracts held either directly with the health authority or PCT, through a subcontract to the NHS trust that owns and manages the site. The flexibility of the service and the integration achieved makes recording and accountability less precise than they would be for a single provider. For in-patient and out-patient services, many use systems designed for acute hospitals, which are not considered to be tailored to the needs of local hospitals and the types of care offered.

Information systems are not well developed through the various departments, and many are still on manual systems for recording activity.

PCG/Ts requiring information on activity, outcomes and costs in order to assess the outcomes, accord priorities and plan the service are often trying to do so on a limited diet of information. In many hospitals there is not an information culture. PCTs will want to make informed decisions about local hospitals, both in their commissioning role and as potential providers.

Case study

The Scottish Association of Community Hospitals has been working with the Scottish Office to design a specification for an integrated information system for community hospitals. This has been developed through the creation of a user requirement document, and validated through a pilot at Hawick. The shared information system continues to be developed, with the support of enthusiastic GPs in Nairn and Brechin. The ambitious project is taking into account community and primary care information systems, as well as health and social work systems. It is hoped that the final product will provide a template for community hospitals in Scotland and beyond.

Investment

The historic shortage of investment in the service and environment produces a legacy which will take many years to redress. Many community hospitals were built in the 1920s as war memorials, and are no longer appropriate in design for modern care and clinical practice. The lack of strategy has meant that these hospitals were a low priority for investment in new services or for backlog maintenance. Subsidisation by local people has proved to be very valuable in this climate. Now that access to local health facilities is a key policy priority, attention is being given to the redevelopment of these hospitals. In some areas, NHS community trusts are reticent about starting a redevelopment programme because of concern regarding their longevity. At the same time, PCG/Ts are expressing a view that they do not want to inherit a service until it has been improved to an agreed standard. In some cases private finance initiatives (PFIs) and public private partnerships (PPPs) have helped to draw in new capital into local hospitals (Jay *et al.* 1999; NHS Estates and Community Hospitals Association 2000).

There are excellent precedents to draw on with regard to constructive partnerships and models that have enabled poor buildings and facilities to be redeveloped. At the time of writing there is a publication pending from NHS Estates and the Community Hospitals Association on models of ownership, development and management which will give further guidance on sources of capital and revenue, and provide case studies and illustrations to follow (NHS Estates and Community Hospitals Association 2000). This has been prompted by the examples of innovation by local people who have campaigned successfully to save and develop their local hospitals. A number have established new organisational structures such as charities in order to do so, as in Odiham (Hampshire), Tetbury (Gloucestershire) and Rye (East Sussex). These arrangements have encouraged new partnerships and have opened access to new sources of revenue and capital. This has contrasted with a number of closure proposals submitted to the Department of Health which have not given evidence of exploring opportunities for wider roles and partnerships. Stakeholders will be encouraged to pursue different organisational models and partnerships such as those with social services, housing associations, voluntary bodies and others. The NHS Executive issued a design guide for community hospitals in recognition of the fact that these facilities are distinct from general hospitals in design and function (NHS Estates 1999).

Case study

In Ledbury, Herefordshire, the 100-year-old community hospital has been identified as a priority for redevelopment because of the age, size and fabric of the building. Local people and GPs had campaigned vigorously for investment in the local hospital. SHAW Homes will be undertaking the redevelopment of the hospital, promising a revenue neutral impact on an improved facility. SHAW Homes are working in partnership with Hereford Health Authority and the local GP practice.

Clinical practice

Demonstrating compliance to standards and consistency with so many clinical medical practitioners has been a challenge. GPs are the independent practitioners with the lead responsibility, but they operate outside NHS provider trust management boundaries. A clear clinical direction from so many medical interests, including all local GPs and visiting consultants, has been problematic to achieve. Mechanisms are now in place to assist with this. In particular, the development of care pathways has helped to provide a guide to co-ordinating managed care. The increase in nurse-led services and the creation of protocols and guidelines for nursing and medical staff is already having a benefit. PCTs will want to be satisfied that safe and appropriate care is given within agreed standards.

The original work by Dr Charles Shaw on setting standards for clinical practice was described by Julia Cumberledge as the most comprehensive publication of its kind on the role and functioning of community hospitals (Shaw *et al.* 1988). Baroness Cumberledge commended it to health authorities and managers as an extremely useful tool in evaluating their contribution.

Case study

The Hospital Accreditation Programme (HAP) was designed for community hospitals by Dr Charles Shaw. It was piloted in the South-West region and is now a UK-wide system, covering community hospitals and private/independent hospitals. HAP is a voluntary system, and standards are set with agreement of the Royal Colleges. Tewkesbury Hospital, for example, achieved a three-year accreditation for its hospital for achieving standards in its services which include a busy operating theatre, a minor injuries department, clinics and wards.

Equity and access

The tensions between equity and access are key considerations for new primary care organisations. PCG/Ts are typically of a size which means that they could include GP practices that have access to a community hospital as well as those which do not. In terms of commissioning, and providing, there is a concern that these facilities distort the revenue envelope of the health economy, and that they take a disproportionate amount of management time and attention. Those GPs in practices whose populations do not benefit from a community hospital are often pressing for an equitable service for their patients. A lack of the kind of parity defined in Chapter 4 is a contentious issue, creating a tension with the requirement on new PCTs to address both health inequalities and improve access to local healthcare. In some areas, alternative models of community hospital services and intermediate care are being developed. These include the use of nursing homes, domiciliary models of care, and community teams.

Access may be defined by geography, transport, referral and admission routes, patient flows and physical access. PCTs should be addressing all aspects of access and equity to ensure that the population gains overall benefits from this resource.

Case study

The Arun PCG has two community hospitals within its catchment area, and has instigated a review of the services with a view to future investment. For a number of years it has been expected that one of the hospitals would need to close, with all services being consolidated on to one site. This could be justified on the grounds of resource efficiency, such as for finance, staffing and equipment. An alternative plan from the PCG is emerging which would result in one centre developing as an intermediate care unit incorporating the in-patient beds, with the other hospital becoming a community resource centre incorporating ambulatory care. Although the hospitals are only three miles apart, local people have campaigned to make a case to retain both hospitals on the basis of access and equity.

Resources

The lack of financial and management resources is a historic position for many local hospitals, which were not considered to be part of the overall healthcare system. Proposals to close community hospitals are usually made on the grounds of cost savings, and the lack of management resources has meant that there is not the information or evidence available at present to help to make an informed decision.

Case study

Hoylake Cottage Hospital in Merseyside was planned for closure, and a new charity was formed to take on its ownership and management. The health authority was committed to a reduced level of revenue, and the charity enhanced this through the provision of nursing home beds. The charity invested in the building and has been responsible for improving the environment whilst retaining the spirit of the cottage hospital. The GPs continue to support the hospital, and these are plans for developing the day services and intermediate care beds.

Conclusions

New NHS PCTs face a number of challenges and opportunities both within their commissioning roles and also as extended providers of healthcare. Many

PCG/Ts are already embracing the intermediate care agenda and national policy direction, and are focusing attention on maximising the role and contribution of their local hospitals. Where this is being carried out with local people, working in partnership with associated organisations, and tackling the wider health and social care agenda, this is likely to be highly productive. PCTs as new organisations are adopting a new perspective on health, and are being encouraged to be innovative. There are many examples throughout the UK whereby the health and wellbeing of local people may be enhanced by the provision of a locally accessible community hospital service, working as an integral part of the wider healthcare system. Local people already see these facilities as valuable community and social assets, and can contribute in a number of ways to helping to achieve the PCT agenda for improving health for current and future generations.

References

Community Hospitals Association (1999) *Directory of Community Hospitals* (2e). CHA, Bristol.

Community Hospitals Association and Department of Health (pending) *Innovations and Best Practice in Community Hospitals.* Bristol and London.

Department of Health (2000) *Shaping the Future NHS – long term planning for hospitals and related services.* Department of Health, London.

Higgins J (1993) *The Future of Small Hospitals in Britain* (occasional paper). University of Southampton Institute of Health Policy Studies, Southampton.

Humphrey I *et al.* (1996) *Community Hospitals in Wales – the future.* Welsh Office, Cardiff.

Jay T *et al.* (1999) *Gloucestershire Study – appropriate use of community hospital beds.* www.glos-health.org.uk/bed%20study/Title.htm

Meads G, Killoran A, Ashcroft J and Cornish Y (1999) *Mixing Oil and Water.* HEA Publications, London.

NHS Estates (1999) *Design Guide – the design of community hospitals.* Department of Health, Leeds.

NHS Estates and Community Hospitals Association (2000) *Models of ownership of Community Hospitals.* Department of Health, Leeds.

NHS Executive (1999) *The NHS Performance Assessment Framework.* Department of Health, Wetherby.

Ritchie DL (1996) *Promoting Progress – Community Hospitals in Scotland.* University of Aberdeen, Aberdeen.

Secretary of State (1997) *The New NHS: modern, dependable.* Department of Health, London.

Secretary of State (2000) *The NHS Plan.* Department of Health, London.

Shaw C, Hurst M and Stone S (1988) *Towards Good Practices in Small Hospitals — some suggested guidelines.* National Association of Health Authorities, Bristol.

Steiner A (1999) *Intermediate Care: a conceptual framework and review of the literature.* King's Fund, London.

Vaughan B and Lathlean J (1999) *Intermediate Care Models in Practice.* King's Fund, London.

CHAPTER 8

Balancing bigger budgets

Robert Moore

GPs collectively now decide where to fund services.[1]

What is the budgetary framework of a PCT?

Primary care trusts (PCTs), whether at level 3 or 4, have substantial budgets to manage. If they are to be seen to be successful they will have to demonstrate an ability to manage these budgets in a way that can satisfy all their stakeholders, and meet the tests for more efficient resource utilisation as described in Chapter 3.

All PCTs have a 'unified budget', incorporating the previously separate NHS funding streams of:

- Hospital and Community Health Services
- prescribing expenditure by GPs and some community nurses
- GP practice infrastructure developments including premises, staff and IT (which would previously have been funded from health authorities' General Medical Services cash limited budgets).

By cutting through the artificial barriers that have been erected between hospital referral budgets, prescribing budgets and GP practice infrastructure budgets, PCTs now have more flexibility over how they deploy their resources. In summary, the policy for PCTs is that:

> By virtue of their size and financial leverage, they will have far greater ability to shape local services around patients' needs. (Secretary of State 1997)

However, despite this apparent flexibility, it is already clear from our experience in the first 'wave' that PCTs will still encounter significant tensions in managing these budgets.

---

[1] *NHS Plan* 2000: 10.7

Budgetary tensions

The first of these relates to how the budgets have been calculated. All PCTs have a *target* budget based on a weighted capitation formula, i.e. based on the perceived needs of the population within the PCT and taking into account such factors as deprivation and morbidity. However, this target budget is not likely to be the *actual* budget received by most PCTs, which will, in the majority of cases, be based principally on historical usage of resources.

The result will be a balancing up, with those above their weighted capitation share receiving less growth in future years than those below. Tensions arise for those PCTs who, aware of needs unmet, will nevertheless have to plan for less year-on-year improvement in resources. Those PCTs below target will have to wait to receive their 'fair share' of the total pot even though they may have already identified major gaps in current provision.

The recently published National Plan (Secretary of State 2000) makes a great play of targeting future resources towards those areas with the greatest deprivation but the interim period will still have to be managed. The lessons of past NHS experience during the 1990–95 internal market and the previous application of the research allocation working party (RAWP) formula is that achieving a 'level playing field' in budgetary terms always takes far longer than central plans anticipate. One reason for this is the tension that inevitably pervades the relationship between equity of access and equity of funding. Many PCTs are highlighting socio-economic grounds in their argument for additional resources to properly tackle the issue of access within primary care. Any weighted capitation formula for allocating resources suffers from close scrutiny at the lower levels, which is exactly where PCTs are expected to make things happen. PCTs will carry out needs assessment for their populations taking into account social as well as health issues. Any gaps in current provision highlighted by this assessment will need to be bridged but resources may not have been allocated on the same basis or criteria, either centrally or locally.

To safeguard practice infrastructure, and also to assuage the concerns of the medical profession, the baseline of resources allocated to practice infrastructure at the commencement of unified budgets has been guaranteed. PCTs are free to increase this baseline at any time but cannot decrease it without prior agreement with all constituent members.

This in itself leads to further tensions. Despite the concerns of the medical profession more 'modernisation' resources have been invested in primary care than anywhere else. Nationally we have witnessed extra resources being used to develop practice staff, primarily through the nursing infrastructure. The introduction of local development schemes to address specific local issues has also increased. Schemes such as those addressing the needs of patients in nursing homes and, more recently, asylum seekers and refugees have been very popular. This situation should not come as a surprise as this has always happened with every large primary care reorganisation. The introduction of family health service authorities (FHSAs) in the late 1980s and early 1990s resulted in the highest growth then seen in primary care development with, for example, a doubling of practice nursing and unprecedented levels of cost rent and improvement grant approvals during the 1989–93 period. Already in the London area two PCTs are looking to reimburse all practice staff at 100%, on the grounds that such staff are a crucial resource for future success. This will result in yet more resources going directly into primary care.

The factors described above will require close management and the development of a true corporate culture in order to make the best use of total resources. For example, how long will PCTs continue to 'compartmentalise' the different streams of the unified allocation? How long will individual practices' expenditure receive budgetary protection? Tensions will inevitably arise between the centralised requirements of the HImP, driven at health authority level, and local intra-PCT level strategies which will have to fight to become part of the stated objectives of the HImP. As suggested in Chapter 3, it is essential that PCTs take a 'whole health economy' stance when looking at what is best. Simply ploughing more and more resources into primary care, even given the drift of current policy announcements, without protecting the viability of the secondary sector will result in a destabilised health economy benefiting no one.

PCTs will be subject to a management cost target relating to their functions and in accordance with their devolved responsibilities, and the requirement to have enhanced arrangements for corporate governance (NHSE 1999). Much negotiation is still taking place to arrive at an acceptable formula. Flexibility in managing cost targets across the health economy as old structures are broken down and replaced by new organisations requires careful consideration. In addition, it is clear that PCTs have received varying resources from health authorities to carry out their functions. This lack of demonstrable overall equity will make the issue even harder to resolve.

Levels of trust

PCTs have been given responsibility for three main functions; improving the health of the community, developing primary and community health services and commissioning secondary care services. There is, however, a difference between a PCT at level 3 and one at level 4.

A PCT at level 3 will undertake all the functions above but will only be able to commission services, not directly supply them. A PCT at level 4 will bring together commissioning and primary care development with the provision of community health services.

In practice this will require the transfer of a considerable number of community staff: health visitors, district nurses, school nurses, physiotherapists, etc., from existing community trusts to form a much bigger and more complex organisation. A PCT at level 4 will also have to ensure it can separate these distinct functions of commissioning and providing services when reporting its financial position. There should be no cross-subsidisation between the functions and audit checks will be carried out to test this. From 2000–01, PCTs are required annually to manage within overall resource limits losing the licence of past NHS cash limit arrangements to mask in-year overspends via deferred creditor payments. This resource will consist of the three separate funding streams plus an allocation for management costs. For a PCT at level 4, there will also be the required allocation to cover the provider function of the organisation.

The overall budgetary framework of a PCT is more complex than previous primary care organisations, especially for those trusts at level 4. The flexibilities given by the 'unified budget' do mean that PCTs have the ability to focus resources on prioritised areas for the benefit of the local population. However, constraints will continue to exist, of which the financial situation within the local secondary sector is likely to be the most pressing. Extra resources have had to be ploughed into the secondary sector by the initial PCTs to offset current and residual deficits and, whilst this is intended to clear deficits, past NHS experience would suggest future demands will continue to be made.

The development of 'one stop shops' in primary care will not, of course, be possible without full participation with secondary providers. Plans are already afoot in a number of PCTs to develop diabetes centres to provide holistic care to all patients, as the case studies in Chapter 7 illustrate. Such centres include, typically, diabeticians, dieticians, podiatrists and the provision of diabetic retinopathy all on one site. Patients can initially see all professionals on their first visit with future care responsibilities being determined afterwards. In North Peterborough the consultant in diabetic care from the acute trust has been involved in these discussions and supports the proposals, including the provision of consultant clinics within the new centre. This is a good example of new ways of thinking and the shaping of local services around patients' needs by utilising resources from the different funding streams. Compromises have to be made by all parties but only by undertaking such dialogue will change be possible.

Information management

There is also a requirement for PCTs to monitor non-financial information and this plays a vital role in the overall budgetary framework.

By far the most important non-financial information relates to waiting lists, and, post-millennium, waiting times. PCTs are required to report on current positions in respect of both in-patient and out-patient waiting times. It is important for the PCT to understand the backwards link to referral patterns of GPs within the PCT. One PCT, for example, undertook an audit of all orthopaedic referrals in the early 2000–01 cycle to try and determine the reasons behind the increase in the numbers on waiting lists. The audit highlighted a number of referrals deemed to be 'inappropriate'. This exercise has resulted not only in new protocols being agreed for all orthopaedic referrals but a better understanding of the role that physiotherapists can play in the treatment of some orthopaedic problems.

The role that cross referrals within primary care can play has also been highlighted and action will need to be taken to train interested GPs to undertake work based on particular areas of clinical expertise (the National Plan considers this issue when looking at developing GP specialists within primary care). Is this 'rocket science'? Hardly, but through the understanding of the links between referrals at primary care level and a willingness for all parties to work together, a new system has been developed which will hopefully tackle the waiting problems in this orthopaedic specialty. It is usual for waiting times to be analysed by main providers and to be sub-divided by specialties. In similar ways the PCT can identify specific areas of concern and agree an action plan for correcting any deviations from the plan.

For a PCT at level 4, the monitoring of workforce planning and sickness rates is also a crucial requirement to ensure the retention and recruitment of a skilled workforce that will be able to support the provider function of the organisation.

What can be learnt from others?

The introduction of PCGs, and, from 1 April 2000, PCTs, placed more responsibility with primary care, and primary care practitioners, than ever before. This could be seen as an onerous responsibility and certainly not one to be taken lightly. However, this is not new territory, others have gone down this path before, and PCTs will need to look closely at learning from what others have done. In terms of overall financial management responsibilities there are some specific areas that need to be covered.

Corporate governance

PCTs must demonstrate that they have effective management systems in place that safeguard public funds. It is crucial that managers at all levels have clearly agreed objectives with well defined responsibilities for making best use of resources. Primary care has not been renowned in the past for having robust systems in place for identifying and clarifying objectives and with PCTs this will have to change. All managers should be appraised and held to account for the responsibilities assigned to them and this will require a system of reviews that identifies gaps in current knowledge and thus training requirements.

Having a 'vision' that is both shared and understood will be a prerequisite to this and will also inform both local and national agendas.

A good example is the requirement for each PCT to produce a Primary Care Investment Plan (PCIP) to incorporate local and practice-based development intentions within a rolling programme. The PCIP also needs to reflect wider HImP priorities and these may well focus on issues specific to certain areas within the PCT, beyond practice and local levels. For example, premises development is key to ensuring the future provision of high quality care. The PCT needs to have a plan for such development that is shared by all parties. GPs will need to adopt a corporate vision for primary care rather than focusing specifically on the requirements of their own practice. This change may well be difficult for some practices to accept but accept it they must if a corporate style of management is to prevail in the interests of the whole PCT community. Such corporacy is the basis for all the best budgetary principles and practice.

To assist in this process PCTs need to help all practices develop practice-based development plans that can inform the PCIP and link to the HImP and the service and financial framework (SaFF) process. In this way PCTs can aid practices to develop a corporate view of PCT-wide requirements and demonstrate how they can play their part in taking the agenda forward. PCTs should look to other NHS trusts to see how they are structured to deal with this agenda. In turn, consideration of organisations outside of the NHS also needs to be encouraged as the private sector has long experience of, and expertise in, developing corporate financial management. The role of the board within a PCT is similar to that of the board of a public limited company and PCTs could usefully look at some of these companies to see how strategic decisions are arrived at, and more importantly, how such decisions are cascaded down through the organisation.

Organisational structures can play a vital role in ensuring top level information is passed down adequately. Accordingly, PCTs need to ensure a flexible structure to enable the organisation to react quickly and effectively within the current and future complex environments of change.

As indicated in Chapter 3, the availability of information is a key element. Reference has already been made to the link between referrals and waiting lists. PCTs are in a position to use their size to go behind such figures to identify the 'drivers' affecting behaviour and to seek to intervene where appropriate. In particular, National Service Frameworks (NSFs) are a valuable aid for PCTs to show that targets are being met. In order to achieve this PCTs need to be assured that GP practices can provide this information in an acceptable format.

A number of PCTs (and PCGs) have involved themselves in the PRIMIS project (Primary Care Information Services), which seeks to ensure the availability of common health data within primary care. This project not only works with practices to ensure common data input and retrieval but also assists in change management issues required within practices to make this work. The PCT that does not recognise the importance of having good, reliable information will be the PCT that does not survive in the long term.

Controls assurance and risk management

Controls assurance relates principally to internal financial controls and PCTs need to ensure that systems are in place that demonstrate adherence to these requirements. Once again, PCTs should look to other organisations to see how they have developed controls assurance to guarantee that the minimum standards are met. These minimum standards should ensure that:

- the PCT has signed up to the Codes of Conduct, Accountability and Openness
- standing Orders and Standing Financial Instructions are in place
- there is a fraud and corruption policy in place
- there is a register for declaration of interests
- there is an Audit Committee and a Remuneration Committee in place as subcommittees of the board
- there is an adequate internal audit function
- there is a budgetary control system in place
- there is a mechanism in place to facilitate control over the acquisition, use, disposal and safeguarding of assets.

PCTs are required to identify all risks and take appropriate action. The Annual Accountability Agreement (AAA) with the health authority requires this and includes a provision to break even year on year. Financial risks include prescribing costs (especially relevant given the recent problems with generic 'warehouses') and special placements. The latter can be very costly and unpredictable and PCTs will need to demonstrate that mechanisms are in place for dealing with these.

Schemes of delegation

The PCT has to ensure that there are clear lines of delegation that protect both the financial resources of the organisation and the staff, and the public. Any scheme of delegation should be available to and understood by all staff, so that at any one time there is full awareness of where lines of responsibility begin and end.

Budget/management reports

The PCT needs to ensure that information is regularly provided that satisfies the requirements of all stakeholders. Statutory accounts have to be prepared to satisfy the Department of Health, via its regional offices, that the PCT is managing its overall resources in an effective way.

In addition, the PCT board needs information to enable it to take decisions in pursuit of the strategic direction of the trust. Management information of this type is most important to a PCT and every effort should be made to ensure that the PCT has access to all necessary information streams. It is vital for the PCT to have the expertise to interpret data, using techniques such as cost–benefit analysis, to really address issues at all levels and properly inform decision making. The PCT will need to ensure that information systems, especially those within general practice, are brought up to a required standard.

This section has looked at some of the new requirements that PCTs have to fulfil. No primary care organisation has ever had the responsibilities that now face PCTs. On the other hand no primary care organisation has had the opportunities to shape the agenda that are now available to PCTs.

Whilst the current agenda may be new, it is not a new concept and many lessons can be learnt from looking closely at how other organisations, both within and outwith the health sector, have structured themselves.

What can be done about demand management?

In order to address this issue the PCT needs to be fully conversant with the drivers behind expenditure patterns. Waiting lists are one obvious sign of the demands on the system but a PCT will need to gain wider a perspective to manage demand throughout the whole healthcare system. The determinants of health are not just encompassed within the health sector. Poor housing, social exclusion and a poor diet can all contribute to poorer health and, in turn, more demands on the health system. PCTs need to be aware of this and look to improve their ability to identify the factors that contribute to poorer health.

PCTs, therefore, need to ask the following such questions:

- What services are we currently buying?
- What services are we currently providing?
- Is there an identified need for these services and how has this need been identified?
- Do these services form part of our local plans such as the HImP? If not should they be a priority?
- Do these services contribute to meeting national priorities such as the National Service Frameworks?
- What are the main determinants of the demand on the system?

Some of these answers may appear self-evident but primary care has never been in a position to provide all of the responses, and neither has it worked in partnership with other organisations to develop mechanisms to ensure that all of these questions can be answered satisfactorily.

Comprehensive needs assessment, obviously, can play a vital role in informing this agenda. The use of the term 'needs assessment' rather than the more often quoted health needs assessment is deliberate. Any assessment of needs has to adopt a broad perspective and include social determinants of need such as those already mentioned. Only by having this information to hand can robust strategic plans be developed, on which budgets can be based to optimise overall resource utilisation.

There is a specific requirement for PCTs to work in partnership with other agencies, especially local government, and this has been reinforced by a joint Health Service and Local Authority Circular introducing pooled budgets and delegation of functions between organisations (HSC 2000/010). Social services departments are represented on the Executive Committee of PCTs, again emphasising the importance of taking a 'whole health economy' viewpoint. The NHS Plan of July 2000 went further still with the idea of level 5 trusts incorporating health and social services as never before. With this carrot comes a stick with the implied threat of forced mergers should individual organisations be deemed to be failing. It is abundantly clear that PCTs should ensure that all managers have an understanding of the concept of comprehensive needs assessment and mechanisms should be in place to use the information collected in a meaningful way.

Enhancing the capacity of primary care and making use of the new flexibilities around pooled budgets are two areas that will be high on the agenda of most PCTs. This could be particularly useful in the areas of special placements, care of the elderly and intermediate care where the expertise and mutual resources of both organisations can be used to greatest effect. Tackling winter pressures is also fast becoming a year-round collaborative exercise. Only recently some hospitals have admitted that non-elective admissions are already at the same level as would be expected during the winter period. If systems are to be put in place to avoid massive problems over the winter period, organisations will together need to make the most flexible and innovative use of these new powers. PCTs are already best placed to broker the deals required.

All PCTs have a dedicated, expert resource available to them in the shape of general practice and this resource must be used to its full potential. We are seeing more and more use of nurses as an alternative to the medical model of patient care. The introduction of triage nurses and nurse practitioners into primary care has enhanced the capacity of general practitioners to perform other functions. There are a number of procedures which can as easily be carried out in primary care as they can in a hospital setting. PCTs will need to look at all the alternatives, bearing in mind cost-effectiveness and efficiency, to see if by investing more resources within primary care can result in an improved position within secondary care. Budgetary costs and codes need to be adjusted rapidly to respond to and support such changes. This will ensure that this does not allow a 'dumping' of additional work on primary care but a more structured approach to planning to meet the demands of the system. Primary care practitioners need to be properly resourced for increased capacity but at the same time PCTs need to ensure that the secondary sector is not destabilised. This is a tricky balancing act that can only be managed by involving all parties in joint planning and decision making.

Section 36 local development schemes are one mechanism and the recently announced third wave of Personal Medical Services (PMS) pilots provide a further, more flexible, way of achieving this balance; GP specialists are another.

Care needs to be taken, however, to ensure that all staff have the right skills to carry out this work. Skills need to be up-to-date and regularly monitored and incorporate appropriate safeguards. Clinical governance, of course, has a major role to play. If clinical governance lags behind whilst other developments race ahead, the PCT will face unnecessary risks.

The move towards a patient care pathway approach can only work if resources are shared openly and honestly and directed to areas of greatest effect. Making use of both pooled budgets and the unified funding stream to meet identified demand in the system is one way of tackling the holistic agendas for overall patient care. Working in partnership on needs assessment helps set the baseline and standards for future work that will hopefully see an end to blockages which are a result of the system not working rather than the absence of a willingness among individuals to work together.

How can costs and risks be contained?

The previous paragraphs have described the budgetary framework of PCTs and highlighted some of the important issues that will determine the success or otherwise of these new organisations in their management of their (much) bigger budgets.

In a perfect world PCTs will be able to access the information they need to take strategic decisions and have the staff with the necessary skills to take the agenda forward. We all know though that perfect worlds never exist and that cost pressures will arise in the most perfect of systems. PCTs will therefore have to be ready to manage such cost pressures as and when they arrive. How often have we read in the NHS press of another trust being in severe financial difficulties? And how often has this been down to inadequate management procedures resulting in an uninformed board? This sounds all too familiar but unfortunately happens too often to be ignored. Costs and risks can only be contained if management is aware that there is a need to control them. Self-evident this may be but all too often it is ignored. Implementing effective corporate governance and controls assurance will go a long way to ensuring that a framework is in place to properly inform managers of the position within the PCT. However, this framework cannot work in isolation and must be supported by a board and management who demand the right information and ask the right questions. This may well require a training initiative within the trust to ensure all relevant people are made aware of their responsibilities: PCTs shirk these responsibilities at their peril.

There are some particular areas where risk sharing with other PCTs and the health authority could be beneficial: specialist services are an obvious example. There are other areas where costs could be contained by sharing the risk. High cost patients who meet the criteria for long-term care, for example, can result in a dramatic drain of resources. Such patients are also very difficult to plan for. Looking at pooling joint resources and sharing such risks with neighbouring PCTs is one way in which such costs could be contained.

Common information systems, providing standard information, can also improve a PCTs ability to identify and thus contain costs. The history of information technology within the NHS does not make for good reading but the introduction of PCTs brings with it a much more critical need to ensure that the relevant information is available. Access to practice level information on a common database is essential if PCTs are to have the information to inform future decision making. If subsidiarity principles are to apply, PCTs will have to support general practice to bring all information systems up to an acceptable standard so they can provide the information required for both planning and monitoring services.

Mention has already been made of the PRIMIS project, but other ways may be needed to address all of these issues. PRODIGY, for example, is a decision-making tool that can be used for prescribing within general practice. Linking all practices to the NHS net will also enable a better, broader sharing of information.

Can it be made to work?

The agenda for PCTs is vast and very complex. Added to this issue of scale, the pace of change has been such that most first wave PCTs have had to be reactive to demands in order to meet agendas. If these new organisations are to work, a much more proactive stance is required. Primary care will have to throw off the isolationist mantle and don the coat of many colours. These colours will, of course, represent all the partners that have to be involved in ensuring that the provision of services really does meet identified needs.

This presents a challenging agenda but the price of failure may be high for primary care. This may be seen as the last chance for primary care to take control of its own destiny and shape the future NHS agenda. Revalidation is just around the corner and public sympathy with the 'gatekeeper' of health services is at a lower ebb than at any time in NHS history. PCTs need to recognise this and work with their constituents to make these changes as painless, but as constructive and effective as possible.

It certainly can be made to work but only by working together, in partnership and with a complete spirit of openness. Demonstrating successful budgetary control together with more creative budgetary support for improved healthcare and enhanced service developments and delivery, and all that goes with these, represents the best possible way for PCTs to show they are here to stay.

References

Health Service Circular (2000/010) *Implementation of Health Act Partnership Arrangements*. Department of Health, London.

NHS Executive (1999) *Primary Care Trusts: establishing better services*. Department of Health, London.

Secretary of State for Health (1997) *The New NHS: modern, dependable*. Department of Health, London.

Secretary of State for Health (2000) *The NHS Plan*. Department of Health, London.

CHAPTER 9

Developing new organisations: a case study

Elaine Cohen

For too long NHS organisations have been left to sink or swim.[1]

Primary care groups as the harbingers of primary care trusts

Harbinger is a word commonly associated with doom. However, its dictionary definition of 'one that pioneers in or initiates a major change' provides a more optimistic note, and it is used with this meaning in the pages that follow.

Purpose and direction

The current government's stated policy for health services in the twenty-first century is based on achieving the following five key themes:

- improving the health of everyone, and the worst off in particular
- ensuring people get prompt, convenient care and treatment
- delivering excellence everywhere and tolerating unacceptable standards nowhere
- guiding people smoothly through the health and social care systems
- investing public money wisely to get the best results for the most people.

---

[1] *NHS Plan* 2000: 2.26

Its central motif for the organisational developments these require is collaboration not competition, and the phrase 'joined-up thinking' has been coined as a result (Labour Party 1999). In order to achieve these changes, the government set in train a series of structural changes in the NHS in 1997. They directed the 101 health authorities in England, as 'the statutory bodies mainly responsible for planning the development of services and leading the implementation of national health policy at a local level', 'to lead and shape' these developments (Secretary of State 1997).

The central element of these developments was the formation of PCGs which, as subcommittees of health authorities, were set up to act as the initiators, or harbingers, of PCTs. PCGs came into being on 1 April 1999, with the first PCTs becoming operational in April 2000. There were 17 PCTs at this time.

These major changes have followed a decade of comparably significant changes started by previous Conservative governments, for those working in the NHS – the rise and fall of the internal market, the formation of acute and community trusts, the subsequent mergers between some trusts, the amalgamation of district health authorities and family health service authorities into health commissions, and the translation of regional health authorities into regional offices of the NHS Executive. And that is only to name but a few: it has been a period of demanding and unprecedented organisational development.

The pendulum has now swung against the internal market, and some of the changes, but by no means all of them, now have to be unpicked by the new organisations.

This chapter presents an implementation plan which covers the key changes in transforming a PCG into a PCT. It focuses on one typical inner city PCT. Each PCG will, of course, have its own particular set of circumstances. The theoretical framework upon which the plan is based is that developed by Beckhard and Harris (1987) on organisational transitions and managing complex change. Other relevant models and concepts are used to supplement this framework as appropriate. The case study is offered specifically as a simple example of the new NHS drawing on relevant applied research from beyond its normal organisational boundaries.

PCGs and PCTs were introduced in the White Paper *The New NHS: modern, dependable* (Secretary of State 1997) and the intention was that the four levels (*see* Figure 9.1) would allow for local flexibility, in terms of pace and scale of change. One of the government's chief policy advisers in the preparation of its 2000 National Plan, however, assessed the changes as being significant principally for their further shift towards US-style managed care arrangements (Ham 1999):

The aspiration to manage primary care and to achieve closer integration with community health services that lies behind the setting up of PCTs is an attempt to move general practice into the mainstream of the NHS and to ensure greater consistency in standards and services across the country. As such, PCTs represent a challenge to the continuing independence of the medical profession and are designed to facilitate the implementation of national policies, particularly those concerned with the quality of service delivery. (p. 160)

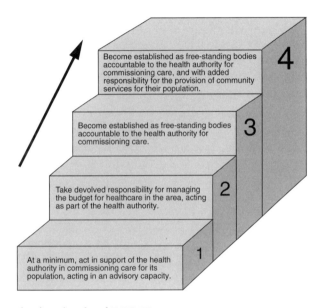

Figure 9.1 The four levels of PCG/Ts.

Background to an inner-city PCG

From the 101 health authorities in England, 481 PCGs were formed. This paper will now focus on one of these, a PCG which is based in central London, and its key stakeholders. The PCG is one of three in the local health authority. It has a population of 105 000, more or less the 'ideal' size for a PCG according to the original central guidance (Secretary of State for Health 1997). It lies entirely within the boundaries of one local authority. However, the other two PCGs in the area both straddle this and another local authority. Community health services are provided by the NHS community trust, and specialist mental health services are now provided by a newly formed large NHS mental health trust which covers three boroughs and six PCGs.

The area is geographically small (no more than two miles across) but it still has pockets of extreme deprivation and extreme affluence. It also has a wide ethnic diversity, including large Arabic and Chinese communities. Within the area are 24 GP practices with 45 GPs (11 of them are single-handed practitioners). Fifteen of the practices were previously part of a fundholding multifund. The practices in the multifund worked in close collaboration for six years of fundholding. The nine practices that combined with the multifund practices to form the PCG had not previously engaged in collaborative working, although the majority of them have worked hard to develop the PCG as an organisation. As the PCG went into its second year in April 2000 the 'them and us' views were fading.

The key stakeholders that relate to the PCG are illustrated in Figure 9.2 below.

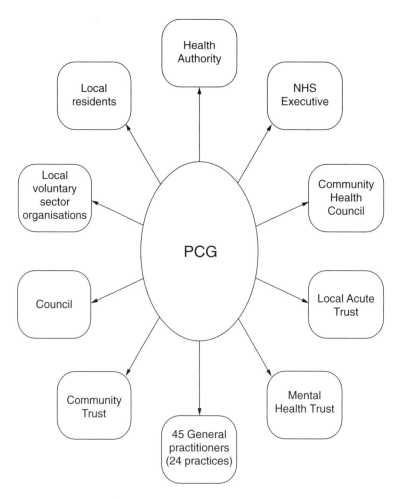

Figure 9.2 Key stakeholders in the PCG.

The organisational change

The PCG operates with a board, the composition of which is centrally defined, supported by its own management team. This team, the composition of which is determined locally by each PCG, comprises a Chief Executive, Finance and Primary Care Directors, a Commissioning Manager, a Finance Manager, a Prescribing Adviser and a staff of six, providing administrative support. The PCG management team operates in an organic way, as the work they undertake is developmental, requiring collaboration and flexible working by all members of the team. This is in sharp contrast to the health authority (of which the PCG is an official sub-committee), which has a

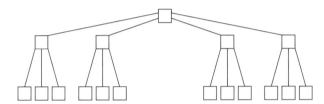

Figure 9.3   The 'mechanistic structure' of health authorities/community trusts.

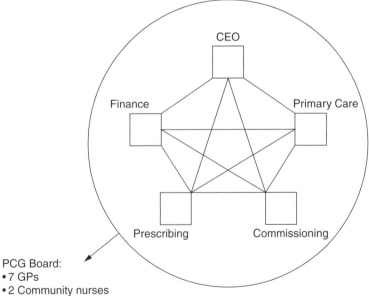

PCG Board:
• 7 GPs
• 2 Community nurses
• 1 Social Services nominee
• 1 Lay member
• 1 Health authority non-executive
• 1 PCG Chief Executive

Figure 9.4   The 'organic structure' of primary group care.

traditional mechanistic structure and approach and also to the community trust. The different structures of these organisations are shown in Figures 9.3 and 9.4.

The task facing the PCG is to transform itself, and the elements of the community trust which currently operate within the geographical boundaries of the PCG, into a genuinely new kind of organisation.

The framework for organisational development

Transferable learning has been an explicit process within the PCG with the approach to the implementation of this organisational change adopted from the applied research in other sectors of Beckhard and Harris (1987). This looks at organisational development in five key stages:

- determining the need for change and the degree of choice about change
- defining the desired future state
- describing the present state
- determining the work to be done
- managing during the transition stage.

The key points at each stage will be outlined and the tasks for the PCG will be described. The model was selected for use because it offered both a clear and simple management process and the means of incorporating both external and internal pressures and priorities so evident in a 'melting pot' situation.

Phase 1: Determining the need for change

Change in the NHS is determined through the interplay of political, public and professional forces, with the relative autonomy of NHS bodies such as health authorities allowing central policy to be adapted and moulded to suit local circumstances. Accordingly the government has decided that all areas of England must have PCGs, although the pace of change towards PCTs is to be decided locally within each region and district, subject to a final completion date of April 2004 (Secretary of State 2000).

In general terms, in an assessment of whether and when to make the change from PCG to PCT status the following factors need to be considered:

- the location and assessment of external pressures for change
- the location and assessment of internal pressures for change

- an assessment of personal agendas of the management and board
- the degree of choice about whether to change.

External pressures for change

The external pressures or resistance come from a number of other organisations. These collectively can be termed the 'local health economy' and are:

- the community trust
- the health authority
- surrounding PCGs
- the local authority
- local acute trusts
- local residents (service users and carers)
- local voluntary sector organisations
- the mental health trust.

Each of these organisations and the other PCG stakeholders (*see* Figure 9.2) have their own perspective on the necessity for change and on the appropriate pace of change.

The community trust, which will cease to exist in its current configuration, is the most affected, although the intended organisational direction of surrounding PCGs is also critical. If all the PCGs in an area decide to proceed to PCT status at the same rate, then community trust changes can be managed across all PCGs. However, if the surrounding PCGs are unable or unwilling to change at the same rate the consequences for the community trust are that it becomes a fragmented and destabilised organisation.

In order to address these issues, effective communication channels between the senior management teams of all organisations need to be established. Large meetings are not necessarily productive, and therefore the following more focused encounters have been set up in the district:

- fortnightly meetings of PCG chief executives and chairs
- monthly meetings with the health authority and all the PCG chief executives and chairs and a series of 'away day' sessions
- a monthly Local Health Economy Forum (chaired by the chief executive of the health authority)
- a working group of the PCG chief executive, directors and the community trust chief executive and human resources director.

In addition to these groups, it has been important to utilise established informal links across organisations to explore the viewpoints of senior managers and other staff. This enables the PCG management team to ascertain the supporters of change as well as where the resistance lies.

Internal pressures for change

The main internal pressures for change within a PCG have come from the following groups:

- PCG Chair and Board
- GPs
- practice staff
- community nursing staff.

Apart from the PCG Board, these groups are less concerned with the 'bigger picture' and strategic benefits of the transformation from a PCG to a PCT and will be more concerned with how any changes affect their business and way of working. The preferred pace of change for these groups is slower – PCGs, after all, have been in existence for only just over a year and practices and the staff working for and with them are just getting used to the New NHS.

These groups are also concerned about how changes will affect them as individuals. Practices are very small organisations which operate as small businesses. As such they are concerned about the maintenance of their own income streams. These are their families' livelihoods. Accordingly, the views and concerns of these groups have to be sought and addressed on a more personal basis. The following consultations have been necessary:

- visits to practices by PCG management team and GP Board members
- open plenary sessions (evening sessions) for all local staff
- 'away weekends' for GPs, key staff members and community nurses
- PCG employment of a community development worker to work with local voluntary sector organisations.

Personal agendas for change

Given the extent to which, as Chapter 2 has vividly indicated, primary care organisations are their personal creations, the individual views of the PCG chair and chief executive are likely to be the key force in determining the pace of change. Those PCGs which have chosen to be the first PCTs usually have GP chairs with a history of innovation (especially in GP fundholding), and a desire to be at the forefront of change. In contrast,

PCGs without this history have often entered into PCGs at Level 1 with a more cautious approach. The PCG in this case study was preceded by a multifund. The strong view of the chair is that the multifund was able to make changes beneficial to individual practices and their populations, and that PCTs, with their unified budgets, can build on these developments.

Degree of autonomy

The limited extent of choice for the PCG has centred around when to change, and not whether to change. The prevailing view of the PCG chair and board has been that the change should be made early, but in a staged way which is under the control of the PCG. The experience of changes in the NHS is that those who are slow to change frequently have less say in implementation and receive fewer financial incentives. In order to utilise and inform the dialogue between all parties, and to demonstrate the local benefits of the change from a PCG to a PCT, Phase 2 of the change framework therefore had to be developed at an early stage in the PCG's lifecycle.

Phase 2: Defining the future state

The definition of the future state, and the type of organisation that it will need, are a critical part of the organisational development process. Without being clear about the direction of travel, there is a real risk of diversionary tactics holding sway. An esoteric vision, or glib 'mission statement' will merely arouse cynicism and resistance in those who will be affected by change.

The government has published a wealth of official guidance on the establishment of PCTs (NHS Executive 1999). This, however, covers mostly functional and operational subjects such as the appointment of the board and executive and the setting up of support systems in human resources and finance. The vision, other than that described in the original policy document, *The New NHS: modern, dependable* (Secretary of State 1997) is left largely for local definition.

Organisational development frameworks of respected applied researchers recommend that as well as defining the 'vision' or endpoint, it is also important to describe a 'midpoint goal' (e.g. Dawson 1996). This should demonstrate how the organisation will look between the present and the future. This is particularly relevant for PCG to PCT transformation, as it is intended that the PCT will not assume all the responsibilities of the health authority with regard to commissioning, nor all the provider responsibilities of the community trust in its first year. The PCG has therefore attempted to draft a 'vision' which describes the fully-fledged PCT, and also defines the various stages and organisational states along this path.

This document has been produced by the PCG/PCT Steering Group (which largely consists of the PCG chair and management executive, and draws on expertise from others on an 'as and when' basis). It contains only outline organisational structures. These do not represent a finished product and during the consultation period should be regarded only as indicative. The 'vision' document has been used as a tool during the compulsory consultation period. It has been shared at all levels with the aim of enabling all staff to see their future role in a PCT. This has allayed some of the fears about the transfer of employment to an unknown and untested organisation. As others in similar situations have discovered, it takes 'many bumps of collective heads' before 'PCGs and PCTs find an organisational shape and way of working that is truly fit for purpose' (Beenstock and Jones 2000).

Phase 3: Assessing the present state

Having defined what the PCT will look like and what functions it will undertake, the next step is to assess the present. Until this was done, no plans around what actions should be taken could be made. The assessment of the present should describe the current relationships between the various parties involved (*see* phase 1 above). This includes both the formal and the informal. The fact that the PCG only came into being so recently meant that much of the diagnosis of the present state was undertaken as part of the organisational development process required to form the PCG itself. In addition, the changes and actions that the PCG has had to undertake during the last year, including the introduction of clinical governance, the production of a locally agreed HImP and a Primary Care Investment Plan (PCIP) have ensured that the assessment of the present was mostly complete.

This constant state of organisational change has achieved the 'unfreezing' of attitudes required by those in general practice, and their growing engagement in the discussions around PCTs indicates a new willingness to be involved and consider what changes will have to be made.

This is not, however, also the case for the staff employed by the community trust. They are aware of PCGs, but have not yet been directly affected by their inception. In order to address these issues, a Nurse Reference Group has been organised by the nurse board members. This group, which includes all disciplines and grades of nurses working in the PCG area, now meets regularly and is undertaking a series of 'away (half) days' which will allow them to explore the changes arising from PCTs.

The PCG has also commissioned a Communications Review with the remit of understanding how the internal and external stakeholders receive information about the PCG. This will also make recommendations of the type of information and the ways in which it is circulated. The aim is to assist in understanding the present and to gain commitment to our future.

Phase 4: Getting from here to there – the transition state

Beckhard and Harris (1987) describe the key points of this phase as:

- determining the structures and management mechanisms necessary to accomplish the tasks
- determining the major tasks themselves required in the transition period.

In the PCG, the first of these tasks is now in place. PCGs themselves have been established as transitional organisations. Their small, organic structures allow them to operate in project management style, and although they are subcommittees of the mechanistic-style health authorities, they have had relative freedom to manage their own workload.

In order to undertake the work involved in establishing a PCT, the process for which has been defined by the regional offices of the NHS Executive, the PCG Board asked the PCG Management Executive to act as the Project Team. In addition to this group, a Human Resources Working Group (*see* Phase 1) was set up. This group draws upon specialist personnel experience in the community trust, particularly in relation to engaging with the various trade unions at all stages of the consultation and development process. These groups together provide the necessary attributes of successful change management or (according to the framework) 'clout', in that they have the 'control' of PCG resources, 'respect' of the PCG Board, and the 'interpersonal skills' that can persuade those who need persuading (Iles 1997).

Phase 5: Commitment planning – getting people on board

It is at this stage that the planned changes will succeed or fail. If the commitment is not achieved then the development will stall. Once commitment is achieved, the various groups and individuals will be willing to work together. Beckhard and Harris advocate a systematic analysis of the various subsystems, individuals and groups whose commitment to the idea is necessary. The critical mass required for each of these groups must also be accurately determined.

In order to undertake this analysis, the PCT project team has reviewed the key stakeholders who have been identified in Figure 9.2. The grid shown in Table 9.1 is a useful tool. Those organisations, or key individuals or groups, who are identified as being highly critical and with high levels of power, but who may be neutral or against the changes, must become the focus for persuasion.

Once the analysis has been done and the PCG knows what commitment is needed, the appropriate techniques should be utilised. The myriad of organisational development techniques is overwhelming to those who are not experts in the field. The main 'families' of techniques are shown in Box 9.1.

The timescale for such a large change as PCT establishment is short. Public consultation documents had to be available by July 2000. The final approval by the Department of Health was made in October 2000.

Table 9.1   Stakeholder analysis

Stakeholder (group or individual)	How critical to success	For/against/ neutral	Power	Critical mass
Health authority				
GP practices				
Local residents				
NHS Executive				
South KCW PCG				
PCG				
Community trust: • Chief executive/ senior management team				
• Health visitors				
• District nurses				
Voluntary organisations				
Local residents				
Mental health trust				

Box 9.1   Types of organisational development intervention based on target groups

Individuals	Life and career planning
	Coaching and counselling
	T-group
	Skills education and training
	Work redesign
	Gestalt OD
	Behaviour modelling
Dyads/triads	Process consultation
	Third-party peacemaking
	Role negotiation technique
	Gestalt OD
Teams and groups	Gestalt OD
	Interdependency exercise
	Responsibility charting
	Process consultation
	Role negotiation
	'Start-up' team building
	Team MBO
	Visioning
	Quality circles
	Force field analysis
	Self-managed teams
Inter-group relations	Process directed
	Task directed
	Organisational mirroring
	Partnering
	Survey feedback
	Process consultation
Total organisation	Socio-technical systems
	Parallel learning structures
	Cultural analysis
	Confrontation meetings
	Visioning
	Real-time strategic change
	Survey feedback
	Appreciative inquiry
	Search conferences
	Quality of work life programmes
	TQM
	Large-scale systems change

Source: French and Bell 1999

Between October and April, board and executive appointments had to be agreed so that the trust is able to go live on 1 April 2001. In all, the PCT plan had no fewer than 306 action points.

Continuous closure

This case study has given a brief insight into the work facing one PCG during the year of transition. The task is large for a small organisation, and the timescale is short.

The project team planning the organisational transformation had no doubts about the complexity of the task. Moreover, they were also aware that, however well planned, it could still come to nothing. The chair of one of the neighbouring PCGs resigned (for personal reasons) at one point and the PCG was unable immediately to find a replacement. This caused some of the GPs in that PCG to express a desire to change PCGs. This would have destabilised their PCG, and put the entire vision of three PCGs back into the melting pot – from which PCT might now only emerge in April 2002 in an entirely different configuration to that which has been previously planned. The importance of ensuring that new primary care organisations continuously appraise and respond to changes in both their internal and external environments could scarcely be better illustrated, with the 2000 *NHS Plan* already signalling a further stage beyond PCTs to Care Trusts (p. 6). The reality for primary care is that transformational organisational development has become a fact of life in the NHS just as it has in the range of sectors from which the frameworks (e.g. Dawson 1996; French and Bell 1999) applied in this chapter are derived.

References

Beckhard R and Harris R (1987) *Organizational Transitions: managing complex change* (2e). Addison-Wesley, New York.

Beenstock J and Jones S (2000) Time to shape up. *Health Serv J.* **110**(5719): 28–9.

Dawson S (1996) *Analysing Organisations.* Macmillan, Basingstoke.

French W and Bell C (1999) *Organization Development.* Prentice Hall, New York.

Ham C (1999) *Health Policy in Britain* (4e). Macmillan, Basingstoke.

Iles V (1997) *Really Managing Healthcare.* Open University Press, Buckingham.

Labour Party (1999) *National Policy Forum Report.* The Labour Party, London.

NHS Executive (1999) *Primary Care Trusts: establishment, the preparatory period and the functions.* Department of Health, London.

Secretary of State (1997) *The New NHS: modern, dependable.* Department of Health, London.

Secretary of State (2000) *NHS Plan.* Department of Health, London.

CHAPTER 10

Making friends with clinical governance

Michael Berridge

Patients have the right to expect assurances about the quality of care that they receive, wherever they receive it.[1]

Introduction

'Off-sick', the end of professional autonomy, managerial control of the work of professionals or a new NHS that truly 'has quality at its heart'? The jury is probably still out, but one thing is for sure; clinical governance is here to stay.

The NHS has, until now, shied away from any comprehensive system of assuring and improving the quality of care it delivers. It is easy to forget, however, that there has been no shortage of previous initiatives to introduce quality management into the NHS. Indeed, there has been such a bewildering array of these attempts that critics have diagnosed the NHS as suffering from a case of chronic *quality initiativitis* (Taylor 1998). Most have been and gone, having had little lasting impact – either failing to concentrate on any one line long enough or treating quality as a 'bolt-on extra' rather than something fundamental to the way care is provided. So why will clinical governance be any different?

Well, *The New NHS* White Paper (Secretary of State 1997) sees the current modernisation agenda as having a life span of ten years and clinical governance *is* seeking to be something fundamental to the way care is provided. It challenges professional autonomy, but arguably any policy on quality always does. The world, however, is changing, and professional self-regulation, once a founding principle of the NHS, seems unlikely to survive the failures of healthcare that appear in the media almost daily. And if these failures seemed mainly to dwell on the hospital sector, then along came Shipman.

[1] *NHS Plan* 2000: 8.29

Clinical governance is an opportunity, probably the last, for health professionals to retain control over the quality agenda. Should it fail, then it is likely to be replaced by a far less attractive system of managerial control. The new quality initiatives encompassed by clinical governance have received the explicit support of such professional bodies as the Royal College of Nursing, the Institute of Health Care Management and the Royal College of General Practitioners. Perhaps most importantly, health service staff *do* care about the quality of the care they provide and, quite possibly, broadly support the principles of clinical governance.

For the new, embryonic primary care organisations struggling to find their feet, clinical governance may seem like yet another huge mountain to climb. Success, however, is essential as the future of these PCG's and PCT's rests on their ability to deliver the quality agenda. This chapter seeks to examine the considerable organisational and cultural barriers clinical governance faces and how these might be overcome. Additional material, drawn from two case studies, is presented to illustrate some of the issues involved in implementation, and is augmented by the author's own local PCG experience in Leeds.

Establishing a new culture

Probably the biggest single challenge for clinical governance is the change in culture it requires – in organisations, in primary care teams and most importantly in individual practitioners themselves. Whichever framework is put in place the fact remains, 'clinical governance will have little impact if clinicians do not feel a need for it' (Rotherham and Martin 1999). A similar theme emerged from the highly publicised scandal involving failures in paediatric cardiac surgery at Bristol Royal Infirmary. Although the General Medical Council (GMC) may create the ethical framework within which the medical profession works, it still takes the doctors to internalise the values embodied in that framework. To establish the right culture of shared beliefs, values and commitment to quality, individual nurses, doctors and other staff need to become internally motivated.

A First Class Service acknowledged that this cultural change is best achieved at a local level (NHSE 1997). In order to succeed, clinical governance leaders will need to engage fellow professionals, share their 'vision' and instil positive attitudes to change.

Gaining the trust of local practitioners will be essential. However, change management theories show us that at times of change, trust becomes the most difficult to establish (e.g. Dawson 1996). Many clinical governance leads have expressed concern that engaging professionals and gaining their trust will be difficult as long as clinical governance is perceived as threatening, i.e. that its main purpose is to 'root out the bad apples' or to police or punish poorly performing doctors. Furthermore, to many health professionals the rhetoric of a 'blame-free culture' seems at odds with a government that is seen by the press as 'naming and shaming' like never before.

Implementing clinical governance also requires a change in organisational culture, both at the primary healthcare team and PCT levels. If the *de facto* leaders of most primary care teams – the GPs – remain resistant to the new messages, then the development of these teams is likely to be slow. For primary care organisations struggling to come to terms with their very existence, vigorously supporting clinical governance may not be seen as a priority. However, without exceptional leadership and a real commitment to clinical governance at PCT level it is unlikely that the cultural change will occur.

Organisational development

In implementing the *New NHS* reforms, primary care organisations face a daunting agenda in terms of their organisational development. In no case is this more so than clinical governance – as one manager in the following case studies put it, 'clinical governance *is* organisational development'.

Delivering demonstrable quality improvements in primary care will be difficult enough, but it must not be forgotten that clinical governance also has a multi-agency and multi-sectoral remit! However, just as clinical governance requires PCTs to develop their organisations effectively it may also be instrumental in that development. Clinical governance has the potential to be a useful (and, in some cases, maybe the only) means of engaging local health professionals and other sectors with the PCT. The same argument is applicable to primary care teams – whether in response to a perceived external threat or simply to demonstrate excellence, the clinical governance agenda may encourage better teamworking and organisational development at this level.

Models of organisational development and change management are outlined elsewhere in this book. The cultural values of the 'learning organisation' that underpin this are required at every level if clinical governance is to succeed (Senge 1990).

Delivering clinical governance

Change does not occur simply because someone has a vision and a receptive culture exists. Attention needs to be focused on the process of implementing change.

Clinical governance builds on many activities that have existed before and introduces some that will be new. It is generally agreed that these components are:

- audit
- education and training
- continuing professional development
- clinical risk management
- quality improvement
- evidence-based practice
- measures for identifying and tackling under-performance.

Within many PCTs, such activities as audit, education or implementing evidence-based practice may already be strongly established. In others they may need to be started virtually from scratch. In either case, these components will all require co-ordination into a coherent programme that will, in turn, need to be integrated with other areas of PCT activity covered by the HImP and related planning documents.

Clearly then, clinical governance represents an ambitious agenda for action which, while needing to be 'realistic', at the same time must demonstrate meaningful progress. The RCGP summarises the situation as:

> The clinical governance agenda, while mainly built on existing activity is large. The pace at which it is addressed will be crucial. Every PCG will need to tread a course between over-optimism and inactivity. We advise setting a pace that ensures that primary care professionals continue to be committed to clinical governance. (Royal College of General Practitioners 1999)

It is obviously not possible to be prescriptive as circumstances and priorities will vary from one locality to another. However, some themes do appear to be emerging.

Audit

Clinical audit is, without doubt, a cornerstone of clinical governance. After all, how can we improve quality if we do not know what we are doing now? Before getting too carried away though, it is worth remembering that the past experience of audit in primary care has been far from encouraging.

In 1989, *Working for Patients* (NHS Management Executive) introduced medical audit as a virtually mandatory process for both hospital consultants and GPs. Additionally, it was wholeheartedly supported by the RCGP who had been advocating its widespread introduction into primary care for many years. Local medical audit advisory groups (MAAGs) were duly set up around the country and were required to assist and facilitate the implementation of audit into primary and secondary care. In reality, official policy guidance on medical audit never contained the words 'compulsory' or 'mandatory' and its uptake by GP teams was patchy. Those practices that chose to pursue the process were enthusiastic in its support, despite (at the time) a lack of convincing evidence that it could actually change clinical behaviour in practice (i.e. completing the loop of the audit cycle). And if such evidence was available, '... it was one thing to show that a group of clinicians committed to audit could change their practice but quite another to show that such change could be obtained from the less committed' (Harrison and Pollitt 1994). Audit has also been further criticised for being the 'private domain' of the medical profession and being rigorously protected from public scrutiny.

Medical professionals have generally been less than enthusiastic in their support of audit, if for no other reason than it can be a tedious and time-consuming task to undertake. Once more, a change in culture is required. More important perhaps, the absence of high quality practice level data and the relatively poor level of IM&T in primary care needs to be urgently addressed.

Education, training and professional development

Obviously, the greatest asset of any organisation is its human resources and a key challenge for clinical governance is to ensure that the professional development and learning needs of its workforce are met. Traditional approaches to continuing education have tended to be fragmented, non-participative and usually uni-professional. There has been virtually no attempt to identify learning needs or styles and the educational agenda has, more often than not, been directed by the pharmaceutical industry or secondary care.

For GPs, the replacement of a reliance on the postgraduate education allowance with more needs-based and reflective methods of learning, based on personal and professional development plans is encouraging. However, as primary care teams and not simply individuals deliver healthcare, the need for team learning must be emphasised.

So often the complaint of primary care workers is that they are so busy 'doing' they do not have time to 'learn about doing'. In addition, such staff as practice nurses, managers and receptionists have often had little in the way of professional development, receiving training on an *ad hoc* basis only when work pressures and finances allow. PCTs could make a lot of friends among their constituent professionals if they were to co-ordinate, facilitate and support a credible package of education and career development.

Doncaster PCG, for example, has devised a monthly educational event that involves all members of all general practice teams. Designated TARGET (Time for Audit, Review Guidelines, Education and Training) it provides protected time by using the local out-of-hours co-operative to allow all its surgeries to close down one afternoon a month. Based around a core educational curriculum, directed by the PCG, it has proved to be a great success with the practices and, surprisingly, appears also to have the unequivocal support of the public.

Risk management

Risk management, although well established in hospital practice is a new concept for most primary care teams. To be effective it requires a multi-disciplinary approach and a genuine blame-free culture, especially if such techniques as critical incident reporting are to be effective. As well as the obvious benefits to patient safety, PCT support of practice level risk assessment and protected time for teams to carry this out may produce unexpected benefits including improved teamwork.

Improving the quality of primary care

Without getting into the debate of actually defining quality in primary care (and from whose point of view), how to measure it would seem to be equally problematic. A variety of performance indicators exist and all are open to criticism. Support seems to be growing for the use of some form of accreditation for general practice. Examples include the RCGP team-based practice accreditation programme, the Manchester Emerging Standards Scheme, Investors in People, ISO 1500 and the King's Fund Organisational Audit Programme. All involve peer assessment of one kind or another and measure the (largely organisational) performance of primary healthcare teams against a variety of standards. The advantages of this approach are that it:

- encourages the organisational development of primary care teams
- develops local ownership and involvement in quality improvement
- rewards practices with the status and satisfaction of achieving something they value
- stimulates practices to improve patient care

- demonstrates to the public that practices have achieved defined quality standards
- may help to identify poor performance.

Further advantages to the PCT are that it provides useful data on health-care provision that can inform future decision making.

The disadvantages are that it:

- may be stressful to already stressed and overworked professionals
- places undue importance on what is measurable at the expense of those (possibly equally important) aspects of healthcare that are not
- may be perceived as threatening
- may actually break down the trust between PCTs and professionals that is so important to the development of clinical governance.

Implementing evidence-based practice

As discussed in detail in the next chapter, a major development in the 1990s has been the emergence of evidence-based medicine, and with it, the current emphasis on a scientific basis for all health services. An essential component of clinical governance must be to integrate clinical evidence into general medical practice.

Over the last few years, primary care practitioners have received a mountain of guidelines on the diagnosis and management of a plethora of conditions. Naturally, there are now guidelines on producing guidelines. NICE proposes to examine all relevant research and repackage this guidance in a more coherent and accessible form. For important conditions a series of NSFs (inspired by the Calman-Hine cancer services model) are being produced, many of which will be relevant to the primary care sector. Where 'best practice' can actually be established, then an important role for clinical governance leaders will be to ensure that it is adopted within their PCTs.

The naive assumption that practitioners somehow access research evidence, evaluate it and then incorporate it into their practice has, by now, become largely discredited. The evidence on implementing the evidence demonstrates that the latter is actually a difficult and complex task. Tomlin *et al.* (1998), in a qualitative study of general practitioners' perceptions on effective healthcare, concluded:

> ... [our] findings suggest that the central assumptions of the evidence-based medicine paradigm may not be shared by many general practitioners, making its application in general practice

problematic. The promotion of effective care in general practice requires a broader vision and a more pragmatic approach which takes account of practitioners' concerns and is compatible with the complex nature of their work. (Tomlin *et al.* 1999)

The problem of changing clinical practice is now firmly on the research agenda and there is consequently a huge body of literature on the subject. A major UK study – PACE (Promoting Action on Clinical Effectiveness) – was recently undertaken by the King's Fund. The final report (Dunning *et al.* 1999) should be compulsory reading for all clinical governance leaders and NHS policy makers. Between 1995 and 1998 the programme set out to explore the issues surrounding the implementation of evidence-based practice, using different clinical topics in each of 16 different sites. The final report attempted to draw together the experience gained from PACE with the emerging research evidence about changing clinical practice and developing organisations. Its final conclusions were that implementation:

- is a messy business, requiring facilitation, flexibility and project leaders able to coax, cajole and drive work forward. One group warned 'be prepared to encounter resistance from unexpected quarters' and another expressed the view that 'progress of the project was more evolutionary and incremental than deadline focused'
- is not a linear task, but rather a group of complex interrelated tasks
- takes time, usually far longer than expected – one group suggested that the sensible thing to do was to 'create a plan and then double the time allowed'
- is expensive, and requires lots of commitment if it is to succeed (Dunning *et al.* 1999).

The evidence of PACE, and the other available research, all suggests that a wide range of interventions can be effective in changing clinical practice, but that a multi-faceted approach targeting the different barriers to change is most likely to succeed.

Identifying and tackling poor performance

Identifying and tackling poor performance remains a thorny issue. Initiatives such as audit, accreditation or the GMC's new revalidation programme may help to highlight areas of poor performance. Recently, however, attention has focused on the problem of 'masking' – where the poor performance of one professional is hidden within an otherwise well performing team. Despite exhortations from the GMC and others, the very nature of the GP's legal partnership (and the evidence of history) suggests that the reporting of underperforming colleagues is unlikely to occur with any regularity.

Tackling poor performance is beyond the remit of this chapter but maybe, through clinical governance and the establishment of a new culture, poorly performing professionals can be identified in the future through PCTs' governance systems at a stage early enough for tough remedial action to be unnecessary.

Case studies

To illustrate the issues involved in implementation, the following section draws on material from a study conducted in 1999 to examine the early experiences of two inner-city PCGs in implementing their clinical governance programme. Clinical governance staff in 'PCG 1' and 'PCG 2' were interviewed and many of the comments elicited have been quoted verbatim – they may ring horribly true with those involved in this kind of work elsewhere.

A number of interesting themes emerged around the sheer practical difficulties of launching a new quality agenda into the local primary care community.

PCG 1

Profile

- Population size: 170 000.
- Description: one of the most deprived areas in the country, scoring high on all indices of deprivation. The population is young, expanding, highly mobile (annual population turnover is 26%) and culturally diverse. These features suggest poor health and a high demand for healthcare.
- Number of practices: 40.
- Number of GPs: 100.

PCG clinical governance team

This takes the form of a clinical governance subcommittee of the PCG Board. Chaired by the clinical governance lead, it comprises:

- PCG Board clinical governance lead – a local GP
- clinical governance manager – a full-time post, with the central co-ordinating role. Line management is from a consultant in public health

but she reports to the PCG clinical governance lead. The current post-holder has a nurse management background as well as extensive practice nursing experience locally
- two further GPs from the PCG Board
- one nursing representative from the PCG Board
- a consultant in public health
- the PCG Board lay member
- the PCG pharmaceutical adviser.

The subcommittee has been given clear terms of reference. Areas of responsibility and lines of accountability have been established. It agreed with the PCG Board a plan of work for 1999–2000.

Current clinical governance activity

The clinical governance subcommittee has been meeting every six weeks since April 1999. Meetings are enthusiastic, lively and well attended. They are chaired effectively, and detailed minutes and action plans are produced. The Chief Executive Officer occasionally attends – possibly indicating the importance the PCG attaches to clinical governance.

Written information on local clinical governance has already been sent to the practices and in October the PCG plans to hold a 'launch day' to market its quality agenda. Locum payments and postgraduate education allowance 'points' will be made available to those attending in an attempt to obtain as wide a coverage as possible. It is hoped that clinical governance leads from most practices will attend – any practices not represented will be offered a surgery visit. The latter option could potentially create some logistical problems as the PCG contains 40 practices!

The PCG's practices have all now nominated a clinical governance lead and in nearly every case this role has been filled by a GP. All practices have been required by the PCG to submit practice plans and these contain much information relevant to clinical governance. It is hoped that this information can be extracted and used to create a clinical governance database. Working with the health authority public health team, the PCG has produced a series of performance indicators that may be used in future to interpret practice level data.

There have been substantial amounts of educational and audit activity in the PCG area for several years, although much of it is poorly co-ordinated. It is hoped that this will be incorporated into the PCG's clinical governance strategy. A local clinical effectiveness unit has already done much work with local practices on the audit and management of major chronic diseases.

Clinical governance topics

- Coronary heart disease (CHD).
- Surgery out-of-hours telephone access.
- Infection control in the surgery.

PCG strengths, in terms of implementing clinical governance

- The organisation takes clinical governance very seriously.
- The clinical governance lead is well-liked and respected locally. He is not perceived as threatening.
- Self-directed learning groups have been running locally for some time.
- There is a strong history of locality commissioning and consequently previous experience of joint working between practices.
- Previous local prescribing initiatives have been very successful with high levels of GP involvement.

Local barriers to implementation

- The diversity of primary care development within the patch ('we probably have the best and the worst practices in the country').
- A very demanding population in terms of need, with extremely high consultation rates.
- Lots of single-handed and small practices with poor premises and poor levels of practice organisation.
- Poor development of primary care teams.
- Many local GPs will be retiring in the next few years and have little interest in contemporary developments in primary care.
- Difficulty recruiting practice nurses, practice managers and even GPs to the area.
- Few nurses have specific practice nurse qualifications and even fewer are nurse practitioners.
- Current lack of practice level data.

PCG 2

Profile

- Population size: 100 000.
- Description: a very diverse inner-city population with areas ranging from serious deprivation to extreme affluence.

- Number of practices: 17.
- Number of GPs: 54.

PCG clinical governance team

Currently a team of one – the PCG clinical governance lead, who is a busy, full-time GP! The PCG are re-advertising for the post of Clinical Governance manager, having felt unable to appoint from applicants interviewed initially. When this post is filled it is hoped that a clinical governance team can be formed.

The PCG have employed a management consultancy to aid their development and intend to use this resource to assist in the implementation of clinical governance.

Current clinical governance activity

All but one of the practices have now identified their clinical governance 'lead' and this one practice is single-handed and currently staffed by a locum. In three practices the lead role has been filled by the practice manager and in the rest by a GP. A clinical governance 'away day' for the practice 'leads' is planned.

A local research group, commissioned by the PCG will apply an ongoing project to the secondary prevention of CHD. It is proposed that this will form part of the clinical governance programme but the details have yet to be worked out. A newly created, local mental health task force has agreed to work with the PCG on implementing a mental health programme but again the exact form this will take is still under discussion.

Clinical governance topics

- CHD.
- Mental health.

PCG strengths, in terms of implementing clinical governance

- The PCG Board has committed itself to appointing a full-time clinical governance manager.

- There has been some degree of co-ordination with other PCGs in jointly developing baseline assessments across the health authority district.
- The practice clinical governance leads 'have at least been identified'.
- The PCG has committed resources to fund the 'away day' and sessional payments to practices for clinical governance work to kickstart the programme.
- There are already a lot of clinical governance-type activities happening locally.
- A new multi-disciplinary training and educational support team is now up and running and resourced by the PCG.

Local barriers to implementation

- The clinical governance lead 'cracking up'. In his words '... this is personally quite a strain and I regret taking up the role – last month I spent 56 hours on clinical governance work, almost all of it in my own time'.
- No clinical governance manager and no clinical governance team.
- The PCG has engaged a management consultancy to provide management support, but for clinical governance this is simply not producing any benefits.
- 'Clinical governance is a relatively new agenda and a lot of time explaining it is needed before people understand what it is all about.'
- 'Practices perceive clinical governance as a checking-up exercise and this creates a lot of negativity.'
- 'The health authority are taking a while to wake up to the needs of clinical governance. Their own agenda is so big it is taking them a while to get to grips with PCGs and clinical governance. They do not seem to understand what general practice is about.'

Discussion

Obviously, for whatever reasons, both these PCGs are at widely differing stages of their organisational development, at least as far as clinical governance is concerned. Whereas PCG 1 hit the ground running, PCG 2 was still trying to make a start – however, it is worth remembering that the interviews were carried out only four months into the first year of clinical governance. The government sees this as a ten-year programme. It is possible that the difference reflects the different level of priority each PCG gave clinical governance during their 'shadow' year. Other factors might be the availability of external financial resources and the amount of pre-existing clinical governance-related activity.

The PCG 1 team is diverse, committed and well organised. They are enthusiastic, but retain a healthy sense of realism about the task ahead. The lay representative is also far from being a 'token' member of the public and is actively involved. The PCG is generally supportive and the Clinical Governance Manager has the central co-ordinating role. The clinical governance lead is thus able to adopt a more strategic role, but nevertheless is devoting much personal time to implementation.

The PCG 2 lead had the author's sympathy – the words 'chalice' and 'poisoned' spring to mind. A local GP, enthusiastic and committed to the new quality agenda, this person has worked tirelessly but with little support. The PCG's decision to 'buy in' management support in the form of a consultancy has clearly not been helpful to the clinical governance cause. It is possible that the PCG views other issues as a higher priority at present.

PCG 1 appears to be making good progress and the team is beginning to plan strategically for the following year(s). Comparing the PCG's progress to the RCGP timetable in *Practical Advice for Primary Care* (RCGP 1999), they are 'on track' or better. While they have adopted the national topic of CHD, their choice of local clinical governance topics is interesting. Both are non-medical and appear to be designed firstly to be achievable (correctly) and secondly to engage primary care staff other than doctors. It is likely that documents concerning surgery answering machines and infection control will proceed directly to the desks of the practice manager and the practice nurse, respectively. As poor team development is an acknowledged problem in the area, this seems to be an inspired and apposite choice.

At PCG 2, until the advertised post of clinical governance manager is filled, it seems unlikely that much further progress will be made.

Both PCGs perceive that 'changing the culture' will be the main problem. The PCG 2 lead thought there would be a groundswell of opinion in support of clinical governance but expressed frustration at the difficulty of explaining the complex new concepts to rank-and-file GPs. PCG 1's clinical governance manager felt that the crushing workload, low level of development and general apathy to anything new in primary care would be serious barriers to marketing the new quality agenda. The huge proportion of single-handed and small practices was also felt to present a problem.

PCG 2 was scathing in its assessment of the help it had received from its health authority. The PCG 1 team were less critical and were grateful for the contribution made by the enthusiastic public health consultant seconded to them by the health authority.

Interestingly, no one interviewed mentioned financial resources as a problem, other than obliquely. The main problem is time. There simply is not enough for the size of the task, especially when combined with a job like general practice. The impact on practices and patient care, caused by time attending meetings, visiting practices and generally getting to grips with clinical governance, was emphasised by everyone.

The lack of support staff, such a pressing problem at PCG 2, was also perceived to be a major problem at PCG 1. The PCG 2 lead feared for his sanity right now and the PCG 1 lead did not think he was far behind.

Conclusions

So, for all the hype surrounding clinical governance is there any reason to expect this quality initiative to succeed where so many others have failed?

Professional autonomy remains a powerful force and is self-protecting in nature. The conundrum of defining quality in healthcare means that different stakeholder perspectives will always result in conflicting ideas of what quality improvement should be trying to achieve. And in much of general practice it remains difficult for anyone to define what quality is at all. Quite how users and carers can meaningfully be involved in clinical governance remains one of its great challenges.

The key message appears to be that clinical governance requires a change in culture – for all health professionals, but doctors in particular. As Chapter 9 clearly illustrates, experience from the field of organisational development suggests that such a change is possible but that it takes time, investment and skilled, committed leadership. The government accepts that enacting its quality agenda will take time but has so far failed to invest significantly in terms of resources or the time and training required to create skilled leaders. Ultimately the true cost – the time and energy spent by clinicians in management roles – will have to be paid for, either by reduced commitment from those clinicians to the change effort or by the NHS users themselves, in lost clinical time.

To a change-weary primary care community, clinical governance has inevitably been viewed with some suspicion. Does the policy quietly aim to achieve objectives other than quality improvement? Is it about increasing control over professionals or simply a means of integrating clinicians into management activity? Certainly, there is an apparent conflict between 'national standards' and 'freedom of local implementation' and the latter is at odds with a government known to have strong centralising tendencies.

Ultimately, my view is that clinical governance in primary care sinks or swims with the future of the new primary care organisations. If PCTs are successfully established then so will be clinical governance and if clinical governance succeeds, so will PCTs.

Clearly, the need to enforce quality and service standards in primary care is critical to the success of the whole New NHS strategy. There is undoubtedly a groundswell of support for these new quality initiatives, quite unlike ones in the past. If PCTs can tap into this and achieve the necessary organisational maturity, then they may find themselves making friends with clinical governance sooner than they think.

References

Dawson S (1996) *Analysing Organisations*. Macmillan, Basingstoke.

Dunning M, Abi-Aad G, Gilbert D, Hutton H and Brown C (1999) *Experience, Evidence and Everyday Practice: creating systems for delivering effective health care*. The King's Fund, London.

Harrison S and Pollitt C (1994) *Controlling Health Professionals*. Open University Press, Buckingham.

NHS Executive (1997) *A First Class Service: quality in the New NHS*. Department of Health, London.

NHS Management Executive (1989) *Working for Patients*. Department of Health, London.

Rotherham G and Martin D (1999) *Clinical Governance in Primary Care: policy into practice*. The School of Health and Related Research, Sheffield University, Sheffield.

Royal College of General Practitioners (1999) *Clinical Governance: practical advice for primary care in England and Wales*. Royal College of General Practitioners, London.

Secretary of State for Health (1997) *The New NHS: modern, dependable*. Department of Health, London.

Senge P (1990) *The Fifth Discipline: the art and science of a learning organisation*. Century, London.

Taylor D (1998) *Improving Health Care: the political, managerial and professional challenges of raising health care quality*. The King's Fund, London.

Tomlin Z, Humphrey C and Rogers S (1999) General practitioners' perceptions of effective health care. *BMJ*. **318**: 1532–5.

CHAPTER 11

Taking evidence-based medicine on trust

Jacqui Barker and Leroy White

Doctors, therapists and nurses will increasingly work to standard protocols.[1]

Introduction

It is generally assumed that GPs hold the same views and beliefs about evidence-based medicine (EBM) as its proponents. However, there is growing evidence that this is not the case, leading to EBM having low impact with GPs. This chapter will explore how EBM can best be supported in general practice with GPs and what PCG/Ts can do to achieve this support as part of their new responsibilities for clinical governance, as set out in the previous chapter.

The chapter will explore specifically the expressed professional values and the views on practice and needs of GPs in relation to clinical effectiveness evidence (CEE) and EBM, and, where appropriate, make recommendations on ways of working with GPs that will encourage them to adopt these ideas into their practice in a way which is meaningful to them. The chapter will develop the idea that EBM in general practice requires redefining, in that it should focus on the decision-making process and not the decision.

What is EBM?

The concept of EBM as developed at McMaster University in Canada is a method of developing the lifelong learning skills and problem-solving habits of medical students. The focus is on learning, keeping up to date and

---

[1] *NHS Plan* 2000: 1.22

recognising that knowledge and performance deteriorate with time. Proponents of EBM are keen to make it quite clear that EBM does not replace clinical judgement or experience (e.g. Sackett *et al.* 1996). Sackett's definition is the one most widely accepted and used by the NHSE and NHS Research and Development (R&D) Directorate. He defines EBM as 'the conscious, explicit and judicious use of current best evidence in making decisions about the care of individual patients. The practice of evidence-based medicine means integrating individual clinical expertise with the best available external clinical evidence from systematic research' (Rosenberg and Donald 1995).

Post-1997 NHS policy – roles for health authorities, trusts and primary care groups

The White Paper *The New NHS: modern, dependable* placed renewed emphasis on the role of clinical effectiveness in helping meet the required improvements in quality and efficiency (Secretary of State 1997). A key policy objective of the White Paper is to ensure cost-effective use of resources. This refers first to the allocation of resources to services for which there has been proven effectiveness, and secondly to the need to ensure services are available only to those for whom it is appropriate, i.e. there is a proven likely health gain.

Guided by policy directives, commissioners of healthcare are expected to use CEE as part of a rational framework for determining priorities for investment and disinvestment.

CEE can form the basis for the development of clinical guidelines which can reduce variations in access to service and improve or maintain consistency in the clinical quality of care. It can also help inform the measurement of outcomes of interventions and services, which in turn allows for the continuous clinical audit and improvement of clinical quality. The much publicised case of James Wishart, involving the significant under-performance in clinical practice of a senior surgeon in a Bristol hospital, and other similar examples recently portrayed in the media, have raised the issue in the public mind and highlighted to clinicians that accountability for clinical quality is no longer just a personal issue.

The White Paper has introduced an emphasis on the need to support and encourage the development of systems for clinical governance within main providers and PCG/Ts. There is a clear role in this for EBM and the use of CEE. Quality and efficiency are now seen as going hand in hand, and clinical and financial decisions are for the first time in the history of the NHS aligned (NHSE 1997). The new National Performance Framework for the NHS (NHSE 1999) focused on six dimensions and emphasised the importance of CEE and EBM in achieving the improvements demanded in 'quality and efficiency', particularly in relation to health improvements, fair access, effective delivery of appropriate healthcare, efficiency and health outcomes of the NHS. This has major implications for PCG/Ts who are required to set up systems for developing and implementing clinical governance. Additionally, there is a role for the use of CEE to aid decision making at strategic levels among PCG/Ts in their new or developing role, as commissioners of services (NHSE 1997).

Specific resources and support mechanisms are being set up to drive the improvements in quality and efficiency, which must be evidence-based and at the same time promote and support an efficient and high quality, evidence-based healthcare system. These are:

- R&D programmes which aim to ensure the provision and dissemination of high quality scientific evidence on the cost-effectiveness and quality of care: a programme of evidence-based development
- National Service Frameworks setting out standards and monitoring for particular conditions
- the National Institute for Clinical Excellence with a role of producing guidelines and audits
- the Commission for Health Improvement to oversee the implementation of clinical governance and provide high level indicators on which to measure clinical quality and effectiveness.

Understanding general practice

Locally and nationally, many GPs have demonstrated some initial reluctance to identifying with CEE and the need to practice EBM. The clinical professions appear not to have been inspired to the same extent or shown the same level of enthusiasm as that displayed by policy, politics and the main stream biomedical research community for CEE and EBM. An understanding of why this appears to be the case is needed.

Decision making within general practice is often viewed quite differently to that of a specialist clinician. The latter is seen to be concerned with treating the specific conditions with which individuals present. The generalist, however, is seen to be concerned with treating the condition presented in the context of the whole person. This includes the individual's medical history, co-morbidity, social and personal circumstances and the practitioner's personal experience of treating this person before.

For this reason, applying CEE to a specialist clinical setting may be considered less complex than in a generalist context, where it may not always be the most important factor under consideration.

What do GPs think about EBM? Evidence from the literature

What is evidence?

GPs appear to define evidence (as opposed to other sources of information) as that produced by randomised controlled trials (RCTs) or large meta-analyses of studies (McColl *et al.* 1998). However, GPs are less likely to give evidence from RCTs priority over other kinds of information in their practice and experiential knowledge is considered more reliable than CEE information by trials (Hannah and Greenhalgh 1997).

Are the questions produced by GPs in their practice compatible with EBM techniques?

Given that the basic approach to EBM according to Sackett and others is to formulate a clinical question, then systematically search for evidence, and so on, the level of questions generated by GPs may be relevant (Sackett *et al.* 1996). It is suggested that the level of questions generated was lower than expected among GPs but more so by GPs in smaller, rural practices compared to urban practices (Barrie and Ward 1997). It is also suggested that to promote EBM more support should be given to GPs on question formulation techniques than on seeking and appraising evidence, and better formulated questions will increase the use of different information sources.

Despite the low levels of questions apparently generated by GPs in their daily practice the information sources preferred by GPs are advice from experts or colleagues, postgraduate education, guidelines or such traditional sources as reference books or *The Drugs and Therapeutic Bulletin* (Kerrison *et al.* 1997; Hannah and Greenhalgh 1997). The preferred source is informal advice from experts. This type of advice has a human element, which allows for the subjectivity of applying rules, i.e. identifying exceptions (Barrie and Ward 1997), which may help to deal with uncertainty.

This has been confirmed in other studies, which suggest the clinical questions formulated in primary care are multi-dimensional and complex. The evidence produced through CEE does not deal with the multi-dimensional nature of questions generated by general practice. It has been argued that one of the reasons GPs seek out information on questions from other clinicians is because they understand the questions as perceived in real life (Hannah and Greenhalgh 1997; Kernick 1997).

Application of research into practice

Decision making based solely on evidence from RCTs, for example, were also found to be difficult, as they do not take into account value for money (Kernick 1997; Gill *et al.* 1996). Drummond (1998) discusses the tension between evidence-based medicine and cost-effectiveness. Advocates of EBM say that it is efficacious for each patient even if it is not the best use of resources. The other is the 'social ethic' of attaining maximum gain for a population's health from a finite budget. A bridge can be built between the two to reduce the tension but for GPs, the lack of cognisance taken by the proponents of EBM that 'it may cost more in the long run' reflects what many see as the policy makers' lack of understanding of primary care.

The application of RCT evidence to individuals can be difficult and involve a judgement about the relevance to each individual. Trial data is limited as it provides an indication of effectiveness for a hypothetical average patient or a general probability for a population, and is vulnerable to the application of the normative political values described by Petchey in Chapter 14. Thus, primary care faces the challenge of interpreting this for individual patients.

Some GPs have felt that sticking strictly to the EBM approach would be unrealistic and the process of question formulation, seeking, appraising and applying evidence would be an inappropriate use of the GP's time (Hannah and Greenhalgh 1997). GPs also appear to prefer to use information which has already been appraised and summarised for them, and think that there should be a standardisation of the way evidence is presented. Many GPs did not understand statistics or interpret EBM terminology in the same way (Barrie and Ward 1997). Although some studies suggest there are GPs who indicate a desire for, or have developed, critical appraisal skills, they are in a minority (McColl *et al.* 1998; Kerrison *et al.* 1997). Studies suggest that GPs' preferences for methods to increase access to information are for increased opportunities for discussion with experts or colleagues and access to personal databases.

One study (McColl *et al.* 1998) concludes that GPs with an interest in EBM should be taught critical appraisal skills in order that they can also lead locally in guideline development and provision of advice. Other GPs felt it was not part of their role and would rather see more patients (Black and Thompson 1993).

GP views on EBM

Studies that explored GPs' views on EBM found GPs mostly to be positive about EBM and the positive benefits it could bring to patient care (McColl *et al.* 1998; Hannah and Greenhalgh 1997), although a level of scepticism about the motives behind EBM was reported among some GPs. This scepticism appeared to be borne not only out of a view that Sackett's version of EBM was to a degree impractical and that the topics were irrelevant to practice, but also in terms of the issue of costs. Many GPs felt there was a contradiction between the policy drive to save money through the application of CEE by reducing ineffective treatments and the potential of EBM to increase costs (Hannah and Greenhalgh 1997).

Meta-analysis and systematic reviews suggest that the most effective activities to promote EBM in general practice are patient-related interventions, outreach visits, reminders, the use of opinion leaders and multifaceted activities (Davis *et al.* 1995). The least effective were identified as audit and feedback conferences and dissemination of written literature events without practice-reinforcing activities. Overall the conclusion drawn is that 'there are no magic bullets'.

A commissioned study in the North Thames Region in 1997 looked at GPs' self-reported changes in practice over a period of a year and the information sources precipitating or informing this change. The study found 31 of the 69 GPs in the study had not changed their practice in the last year. Of those who were able to identify a change to their practice, two-thirds indicated information sources other than CEE from RCTs as those used to precipitate change (Kerrison *et al.* 1997).

Exploring the views of GPs on EBM

A series of semi-structured interviews and group discussions were held with 58 GPs in South London between 1998 and 1999. The interviews and discussion guides were developed in conjunction with a subgroup of the Clinical Audit/Clinical Effectiveness Resource Steering Group. The interviews were carried out in GP practices and the discussion groups were held as accredited 'continuous professional development' events.

What informs or influences daily practice?

The interviews and discussions covered a variety of issues. Responses as to what GPs value most as aids in their decision making revealed both variation and commonality. Variations in views on the role of advice from colleagues and specialist advice were linked to size of practice and the ethos of a practice. Single-handers were more likely to prefer specialist advice than their colleagues in larger practices, who preferred to use each other but only internally to their practice. Those that did not were based in practices where sharing of problems was not actively promoted or where limited time prohibited such exchanges.

Most important was the commonality of views. This revealed a strong feeling among all GPs that their experiential knowledge accumulated over the years, and knowledge and understanding of the individual patient and their circumstance was most highly valued. These were closely followed by continuing education.

Responses as to what was important to GPs in their practice almost mirrored discussions around how GPs defined EBM in general practice as seen earlier. For example, that EBM does not fit exactly with general practice, with its particular emphasis on individual patients, or because, due to the nature of general practice, it is not possible or appropriate to base all decisions on CEE.

> The problem we have with EBM is that its fine for the hundreds and hundreds in the trial, but when you have actually got one [patient] sitting in front of you and she says, 'Yes but ...' her 'buts' are something very real.

> Fitting individuals into evidence-based guidelines can sometimes be dangerous.

> I think evidence would enhance the professionalism but can not replace it, the drive at the moment is that we can be seen to belittle or diminish the role of professionals in the care that they provide.

What GPs are presented with does not often require straightforward diagnosis.

> A lot of evidence-based medicine is based on diagnosis and a lot of the time we don't make a diagnosis.

> [Getting evidence into practice] is a judgement, the judgement is about saying there's several things we might value, there's the CEE but there's also issues around cost, time, resources and so on. ...

Cost is a major issue. If CEE were followed according to the strict rules of EBM, then the costs would be higher. There is a whole range of factors that need to be taken into account but these factors and influences, including CEE, will be given different weight depending upon each patient.

> If they really wanted clinical effectiveness they would let us pre-scribe Nicorette or patches. After all, if we could stop someone smoking the cost of savings in the next 20 years would be vast.

The patients' views, expectations, history and their wider circumstances are seen to be an important part of the evidence. General practice is not always about treating patients with diagnosable conditions. It may simply be about listening.

> The ... thing that dictates your daily practice ... is you get patients coming in with various things but if you don't take them as they are part of their lifestyle, their problems which are all ongoing, then you can't really relate to their clinical problems.

> I think the days of ... the GPs deciding this is what you should do have gone and it's a joint process. [We could say] this is my advice and [its] between us that we decide what we are going to do. [This would mean] having available easily accessible informa-tion in simple terms: what the evidence is for and why we are going to do this. This is helpful in decision making for the patient.

Thus the issues that GPs find important in relation to using EBM in general practice can be summarised as:

- context of practice, e.g. practice is not only diagnosis, patients present GPs with multi-faceted issues and co-morbidity
- skills used in practice, e.g. experiential knowledge, medical training
- influences on practice, e.g. evidence from journals, cost of treatment, patient expectation.

The context of practice has been covered in detail in the previous section. The other issues will be dealt with in more detail below.

Skills used in practice

> You base the diagnosis or decision to treat in a particular way on the basis of your knowledge of that particular patient and your experience of treating that particular condition or whatever in a particular way, you might not necessarily use the evidence, the documented evidence might say something completely different to what you decide to do.

Many of the GPs interviewed concurred with the above quote. Decision making in general practice was seen very much as a judgement of factors, many of which may be subjective or patient specific. For example, the elderly lady with acute arthritis pain who has difficulty sleeping is prescribed an analgesic gel despite the strong evidence on lack of effectiveness, because in her mind it is giving some relief from an untreatable and debilitating condition. Or an elderly lady remains on a particular drug long term despite a practice policy to change to another, not because of CEE but because her husband is terminally ill, and the psychological effects of the change at this point in time will be harmful and stressful.

How GPs view and maintain their professionalism, and their daily practice, needs to be understood in order to make sense of how CEE can be incorporated usefully into it. CEE has a part to play in this, but should not be seen as central or of any greater importance than a range of other factors as described throughout this section. Factors may vary in degrees of importance depending on each patient. General practice has a fluidity to it which draws on experiential knowledge and is guided by core values primarily in the patient's interests but mindful of other factors. Decision-making processes are tailored to individual patients; they are complex and involve a judgement. For this reason very strict protocols and procedures cannot be always followed, since in the professional judgement of the GP they may not be appropriate for the particular patient.

For those charged with developing good clinical practice in general practice, this is important and challenging – not least because it may require a completely radical way of thinking about what the most important aspects of good clinical practice are, from both a practitioner and a patient per-spective, and about how can they be measured within clinical govern-ance. GPs are clear that CEE is an important and vital factor in decisions, but it cannot be the determining factor in all cases. What is important, it seems, is that up-to-date evidence is known and taken into account. This is termed evidence-based decision making, and it has an emphasis on the process not the decision and appears more appropriate for general practice (Greenhalgh 1996).

Influences on practice

Improving the GP–patient relationship and managing patient expectations

Aspects which emerged from the interviews were the need to consider not only how to change the mindset of GPs in relation to using more evidence in their practice, but also the importance GPs placed on patient expectations and the need to work with and educate patients in this area.

It was suggested that simply to work with GPs to promote the use of CEE was not enough because patient expectation was such a strong influence on decisions. It was felt quite strongly that work needed to happen with both groups. As one GP quoted:

> It's about sharing with patients, isn't it? You can actually say, well this is what the research is saying – this suggests that this is the best treatment and these are the risks in doing this or that – that way it's not just me making the decision. So you can leave it to the patient once they have all that evidence.

The provision of good patient information on conditions and evidence was important, as GPs did not have the time to explain everything. An education campaign for patients in the area of new evidence on old or new treatments was felt to be important to manage patients' expectations.

Another aspect was the positive view GPs had of the potential role of CEE if it was shared with patients. It was acknowledged that some patients are not responsive to discussions of the CEE of treatments, particularly if these culminated in their not getting the treatment they wanted, and that there were constraints on time available to spend discussing these issues with patients. However, despite this, sharing CEE with patients was still seen to be a potentially effective way of managing patient expectations. This also involves sharing the responsibility for decisions and uncertainty with patients, where appropriate. Other benefits were identified as improving patient compliance, increasing patients' ability to manage their condition better, supporting shared decision making and shared risk, through all contributing to a better quality GP–patient consultation.

The issue of limited available time to share information with patients highlights the importance to GPs of having easily available information to give to patients, to supplement what they offer them in the consultation.

In summary, it was felt that what was needed to promote the full value of CEE in practice was an openness from GPs to share this information with patients, and to tackle patient expectations with patient education and information. It was felt this should be heavily supported by: national and local patient education campaigns; work to encourage GPs to change their mindset on the role of patients; further external reinforcement from a well informed and conscientious media, who are mindful of the implications of their reporting; and, finally, recognition that there will always be patients who are not responsive to either listening to the evidence or sharing decisions.

In addition to the need to target patients with education, some GPs felt that variation in clinical practice among specialists within acute settings also had an effect on the ability of the GP to apply evidence to their practice. For example, this applies to the treatment of tonsillectomy or to grommets as these are areas in which parents often have expectations for treatment, which, however, may be felt inappropriate by the GP.

Specialist prescribing was also an issue. GPs felt that often specialists wrongly assumed or expected GPs to be up to date on the evidence and use of new drugs, and this was often not the case. GPs often felt ill-equipped without specialist knowledge or up-to-date information on how to manage certain patients.

Dealing with clinical challenges in daily practice

In daily practice most GPs did not appear to search for or use evidence productively to deal with clinical challenges or problems. They usually sought advice from colleagues in dealing with daily problems. There were some exceptions to this, in particular in the use of dermatology reference books, the prescribing formulary, *The Drugs and Therapeutic Bulletin*, and specific general reference books that GPs said they trusted and had been using for some time.

The idea of developing questions within practice and then going to search and critically appraise the evidence was not something that appealed to the majority of GPs, although a minority expressed some interest in developing better critical appraisal skills, while others wanted someone else to do the 'finding out' for them, e.g. a researcher or librarian.

Developing practice policies and protocols

Evidence-based practice policies were particularly helpful in reducing GP variations in practice and improving consistency in patient care. They had the added effect of preventing patients from 'playing one GP off against another' in order to get what they wanted in the way of treatment. For most GPs such tools appeared not to threaten but rather support their practice. Given that GPs' priorities appeared to be to reduce their workload, save money and improve patient care, protocols based on CEE which help achieve these were felt to be valuable. Policies and protocols were also felt to have a useful role in managing patient expectations. Ownership by GPs was still, however, felt to be vitally important. It was considered that these protocols and policies should not be imposed, not only because of the limitations of applying evidence in practice as discussed earlier, but also because GPs valued their professional independence and integrity and do not like being told what to do.

Incentives, therefore, were viewed much more positively than penalties, and this is discussed at more length in a later section of this chapter.

How do GPs keep up to date and what influences them to change or vary their practice?

Key ways GPs referred to as methods of keeping up to date or learning of new treatments or CEE were as follows.

- *Continuing education* was mentioned by many GPs as a valuable source of up-to-date information. It provided an opportunity for GPs to: discuss and exchange views with colleagues on practice; explore ideas on new treatments or practice; add to or reaffirm what GPs may have already read about or heard; and initiate interest in developing practice guidelines.
- *Specialists* were seen by some GPs to be a source of knowledge and they referred to learning through correspondence with specialists in order to corroborate the new evidence which GPs may have read about or heard about from other sources.
- *The public health department* acts as an impetus for change or modified practice in relation to drugs and treatments proven to cause or suspected of causing harm. This is likely to be supported further by media coverage, and patient concerns and expectations.
- *Drug company representatives* and the evidence they presented were considered by all GPs to be lacking in rigour or representativeness. However, it was also acknowledged that, although the information they presented had to be taken with a very large pinch of salt, it still did have influence on their practice. Information provided is likely to suggest ideas to the GP, raise awareness of the GP to new drug treatments and supplement information from other sources such as journals, colleagues, specialists, etc.
- *Journals, periodicals, magazines and specialist books* were discussed at greatest length as sources of keeping up to date. Most often mentioned as useful/interesting were *The Drugs and Therapeutic Bulletin*, *Update* and *Monitor*. *GP* and *Pulse* were also mentioned frequently as interesting, but also more as political than clinical and therefore not as useful. *Effectiveness Bulletins* and *Bandolier* were mentioned by only a few GPs. Views on these were that *Bandolier* was too 'busy' and not sufficiently focused, while the *Effectiveness Bulletins* were more accessible because they were focused and 'thin'. Journals mentioned as the least useful and relevant were thought to be the *BMJ* and *The Journal of General Practice*. They

were considered to be inaccessible, too academic and too detailed. Topics covered in the *BMJ* were felt rarely to be relevant to general practice and to be geared more towards specialist acute care.

In summary, the role of evidence in changing GP practice is important. The change process itself is a complex one and although described by GPs in this study as 'not necessarily logical' it is quite a slow and cautious process of experimentation and reaffirmation from a number of sources – not least patient outcomes – which can lead to a sustained change in GP practice.

What will encourage GPs to use CEE in general practice and what are GPs' preferences for support locally?

The uses of CEE in general practice were felt to be: keeping up to date, informing audit, stopping and restricting treatments, developing good practice guidelines, providing impetus to try or avoid new treatments and respond to individual treatments, managing patient expectations, identifying effective health promotion interventions for the practice, and developing drug formulary. GPs generally felt that CEE was most useful to them when introduced through continuing education and prescribing advice. These were more likely to influence their daily practice, particularly if they covered the common conditions dealt with in general practice such as skin conditions, hypertension, heart failure, etc. Levers for the increased use of CEE discussed were financial incentives and penalties, available support based on the needs of and relevance to general practice, and patient education and information.

Penalties and incentives

Penalties

All GPs felt that the imposition of penalties to encourage and increase the use of CEE in general practice was inappropriate and in turn would not be effective. This was partly based on the importance all GPs placed on the need to have sufficient flexibility to make clinical judgements on individual patients. It was also based on the view that penalties were an imposition that was controlling, potentially insulting, and constrained practice and judgement. The motivational element of such penalties was also questioned. GPs recognised that costs and efficiency were issues they had some responsibility for and many felt they already proved themselves in regard to these. It was uniformly felt that cost-efficiency should be sought in equal balance with improved patient care, but they were wary that the drive behind EBM was primarily to save money. This suggested that penalties, therefore, might be more likely to be based on cost saving requirements than on health improvement or patient care.

Incentives

There were some mixed feelings about financial incentives. A few GPs felt that these were bribery and that there were other benefits that could be incentivised, such as improved patient care and services. The introduction of practice-based counselling and rapid access clinics were given as examples of incentives, alongside anything that would reduce workload and improve care. Others were fairly clear that financial incentives were as important.

The idea of nurse practitioners taking more responsibility for the management of certain conditions as a way of reducing GP workloads was raised by a small number of GPs, who indicated that this was something with which their practice was experimenting. The concern expressed was that nurses did not have the necessary medical training. Those GPs exploring this approach mentioned the use of protocols developed with nurses in educational sessions, all of which involved the use of CEE where available. Despite this, many GPs were generally uneasy and felt more evidence was needed on where this was working safely and successfully.

Preferences for local support

GPs were asked to rank the following ways of supporting the use of CEE in general practice (options A to G). If they ranked an option as being the most, or the second most, helpful approach then we considered that to represent 'strong support'. Similarly, if an option was the least, or second least favoured approach we considered it to have 'no support' (Table 11.1).

The findings from the ranking suggest that a range of methods would be required to meet different preferences of GPs. A majority consensus was apparent in the responses to two of the options. Work with the primary care team was not well supported. Paper-based help overwhelmingly received most support. Those who did not want paper-based help seemed more likely to support the personal help option. Those who were in support of electronic help were also more likely, it seemed, to be interested in the GP EBM group.

Table 11.1 Preferences for local support

Support option	A Paper-based help	B Electronic information	C Training and education	D Personal help	E Piggyback	F A GP EBM group	G Work with primary care team
Strong support	73%	36%	5%	32%	18%	23%	0%
Moderate to little support	13%	28%	73%	50%	68%	45%	45%
No support	14%	36%	22%	18%	14%	32%	55%
Total	100%	100%	100%	100%	100%	100%	100%

Training and education in critical appraisal skills received little strong support, and nearly one in four GPs gave it no support. However, the majority of GPs gave it 'moderate to little' support, suggesting some interest but perhaps not as a priority or first choice.

Using solely the data from the ranking exercise, in isolation the most support was for paper-based help (86%) and piggybacking onto continuing education (86%). Both of these are available currently, albeit in ways that GPs' comments and discussions suggested could be improved upon.

The next most supported options were personal help (82%) and training and education in accessing evidence and appraising it (78%). These were followed by a GP EBM group (68%) and electronic information (64%), and work with the primary care team (45%).

The findings from the interviews and discussions reflected the findings of the ranking exercise, showing that, despite the plethora of paper-based information GPs currently receive, the majority, with a small minority exception, still favour this approach. However, GPs were also able to expand on how the paper-based help could be delivered more effectively.

A newsletter which focused on one topic and collated all the up-to-date evidence on the most appropriate management of a condition common and relevant to general practice, written in a summary style, highlighting key points for GPs with differential diagnosis, responses and lengths of treatments, etc. was all felt to be attractive for GPs. A question and answer section was favoured too, based on real questions the GPs may have put to the GP adviser.

Further needs

Continuing educational meetings with specialists

This was the other firm favourite which came out as having even stronger support in the discussion. Again there are some clear ideas on how they could be improved and what factors should be taken into account when organising them. Many of these were similar to those to be taken into account when producing a newsletter, although there were some ideas specific to educational meetings.

The meetings should be focused on one topic with some relevance to general practice and not be too scientific in their presentation. It is important to allow for some dialogue between specialist and presenter through questions and discussion, but also some debate between GPs. Bringing patients as case studies seemed to be favoured, and the local Dermatology Club was referred to by a number of GPs as good practice in continuing education.

How up to date specialists were was felt to vary and not all were considered particularly adept at delivering continuing education events, as this was felt to be a skill not all possessed. Both of these points were felt to be very important considerations for those organising such meetings. A co-ordinated approach to educational events with specialists was suggested in order to ensure a larger proportion of GPs had the opportunity to participate and be updated and also to consolidate some of the learning. This might involve the topic of the newsletter covering the same topic as the educational meeting, with the questions included in the newsletter's Q&A section based on questions raised at the educational meeting. Another suggestion was that there should be more than one educational meeting on the same topic. Finally, GPs suggested that the newsletter or topic guide should be on one side of the paper, and that something to file it in should be provided.

It was recognised that, alongside having a range of different methods to cater for a range of preferences, it may also have to be accepted that at present there will be a small number of GPs who will not be interested in any. In future, PCTs, of course, may not be willing to offer this acceptance.

Training and education in critical appraisal skills

This gained little strong support and three times as much 'no support' response. However, the majority of GPs gave it some support and this, to an extent, was reflected in the discussions. It was felt to be a good idea but not a priority, not first choice, something they would like to do but possibly in the future. Others were clear they did not want that kind of help, they did not want to search the literature and then critically appraise it. A minority were keen to pursue critical appraisal approaches.

Pharmacy advice

This was felt to be something that was valuable in that it not only provided some information on new drugs but, importantly, it helped deal with the plentiful information and persuasion from drug companies on new treatments and management, recognising that sometimes the way or treatment that has always been used or followed is still the best and most effective. This advice was felt to be reassuring for GPs.

Individual patient problem solving was definitely a favourite of about a third of GPs. There were some different views and concerns expressed about this type of service. Some felt a telephone advice line would be most useful for information on drugs, treatments, etc. Others felt that there were risks associated with this, particularly in relation to accountability and litigation. Some felt a service which could be faxed, or telephoned, for information on the latest evidence on a particular treatment or condition, with a response to be provided within the same day or a few days, would be very useful.

Other GPs felt that this would not offer them anything different from what their colleagues could offer them in the way of advice or what a call to a specialist could achieve.

Online discussion on latest evidence and practice was suggested by two of the younger GPs, as was the idea of an up-to-date (annual) CD-ROM A–Z of conditions and treatments giving information on best treatments, treatment length, etc.

Patient education campaigns

Most GPs described patient expectation as a possible barrier to the use of evidence, particularly with those patients who perhaps have a clear idea about what they feel they need. Ironically, many of the same GPs also saw CEE, if shared with patients, as something which could rationalise expectations. For this to be realised, however, it was felt quite strongly that education for patients on the issue of clinical effectiveness and appropriateness should be co-ordinated centrally, and that campaigns to promote better patient understanding on the ineffectiveness of treatments for common conditions was needed. GPs felt that they could not take on the full responsibility of patient education within the limited time of the consultation.

This type of campaign also needed to be supplemented by patient information on the clinical effectiveness of certain treatments alongside how to manage a condition, how and when to use GP services appropriately, and how to treat minor ailments and injuries themselves. It was felt this would be particularly helpful for new treatments, or where new evidence indicated current treatments were ineffective. This patient information would help GPs apply evidence to their practice more easily, particularly for those conditions for which patient expectations existed or had been raised by press coverage, etc.

Topic-based leaflets which could be used with patients detailing the latest evidence on particular conditions were also felt to be a very useful local support, particularly in dealing with patient expectations and helping encourage more involvement in care.

Other suggestions

GPs were asked to consider the kinds of support they felt the evidence-based practice adviser might usefully provide to GPs. Facilitating discussion and debate, linking with educational programmes, working with and supporting individual practices were all mentioned as useful activities for this post-holder. There was a sense that GPs were feeling the need to keep up to date and wanted to be more aware of current evidence to apply to their practice and ensure that their practice is streamlined with other colleagues and practices. There were concerns that this was time-consuming and not always possible owing to other commitments. The support for critical appraisal but without priority was an example where GPs were interested but needed to prioritise their time.

Ways in which learning could be best supported locally were felt to be those which could build on existing resources but improve them considerably. It was also felt that any programmes should start small and develop or evolve, based on what GPs want, and that large amounts of money should not immediately be spent on any one support technique but on co-ordinating approaches with a few district-wide topics.

Conclusions

GPs found that CEE was important in clinical decision making but not always the most important factor. It was seen to have some very practical limitations, particularly in that evidence frequently changes or that treatments can become fashionable, while for many interventions or conditions evidence is not available. Owing to the nature of general practice, it is not always possible or appropriate to base all decisions solely on evidence and there are other factors which are equally, and potentially more, important.

The GPs seemed to want the proponents of EBM and NHS policy to recognise that:

- CEE is not paramount in general practice as it has practical limitations and may not always be available
- it can only ever be one factor in the decision-making process for each patient because of the nature of general practice
- topics need to be relevant to general practice
- evidence-based practice should be monitored on the decision-making process and not the decision
- patient involvement should not be the sole responsibility of the GPs and needs to be resourced by the PCG/Ts.

A GP's work is not as straightforward as making a diagnosis. Experimentation and managing uncertainty is also seen as something central to general practice. The decision-making processes in a GP's daily practice, i.e. how

they deal with daily clinical problems and how they maintain their professional knowledge base, need to be understood in order to make sense of how
clinical effectiveness evidence can be incorporated usefully into practice.

Clearly, for GPs, having an evidence base to decisions is important. Their
argument is that the limitations of CEE and the individualised and complex
nature of the problems that general practice deals with mean that it should
not be paramount in decision making. In general practice, decision-making
processes are tailored to individual patients; they are complex and involve
judgement. Factors may vary in degrees of importance, depending on each
patient. General practice has a fluidity to it, which draws on experiential
knowledge and is guided by core values, primarily in the patient's interests,
but mindful of other factors which may include costs. For these reasons
very strict protocols and procedures cannot be always be followed.

The research reported in this chapter suggests that the following work
with GPs be carried out as part of a PCG/T's local strategy to clinical governance in primary care:

- develop a local working definition of evidence-based general practice
  (EBGP) based on the findings of this study and validated and agreed
  locally by GPs
- develop a strategy for local support activities to promote the locally
  agreed definition of evidence-based general practice. The strategy should
  focus support on creating opportunities for the increased use of CEE in
  general practice, taking into account the findings of this study
- within the strategy a range of methods should be employed, as GPs differ
  in their preferences for support.

Finally, given that GPs do have these different preferences, the following
were broadly felt to be the most useful ways of providing PCG/T support:

- newsletter – to include questions put forward by GPs, drawn from their
  own practice and answered based on the available evidence
- educational meetings – topics to be co-ordinated with those covered by
  other activities in the strategy such as the newsletter and MAAG work,
  and used for the development of practice protocols and even standards
  for clinical governance
- practice protocols – individual practice support in developing these from
  an evidence base. Link in with topics covered in educational events, new
  evidence in newsletter, whatever is being promoted electronically, etc.
- outreach work with practices – this could be useful for developing
  practice protocols, to provide help setting up systems within the practice
  such as clinical problem-solving groups, library access to journals etc., to
  help reinforce and maintain changes in practice, to problem solve on
  organisational issues relevant to promoting the use of CEE

- specialists – better use of communication between specialists and GPs on the evidence base for new drugs and treatments and more information on the aetiology, symptoms and progression of conditions
- patient educational information to be provided to support other activities in the strategy
- evidence-based patient information on conditions should be more freely available to patients and GPs to pass on to patients
- consider carrying out a short review of the available electronic systems which provide access to CEE designed for use in general practice
- any standards developed for clinical governance in general practice should be mindful of the locally agreed definition of EBGP.

This chapter has focused on views of general practitioners. However, for effective clinical practice within future NHS PCTs, it is important that the views of all health professionals are taken on board with regard to evidence and clinical governance, and perhaps eliciting the views and priorities of other professionals in the manner conducted for this chapter would be a step towards achieving this.

References

Barrie A and Ward A (1997) Questioning behaviour in general practice. *BMJ*. **315**: 1512–15.

Black N and Thompson E (1993) Obstacles to medical audit: British doctors speak. *Soc Sci Med*. **36**(7): 849–56.

Davis *et al.* (1995) Changing physicians' performance – a systematic review of the effect of continuing medical educational strategy. *JAMA*. **274**(9).

Drummond M (1998) Evidence-based medicine and cost effectiveness: uneasy bedfellows. *Evidence-based Med*. **3**(5): 133.

Gill, Powell, Neal *et al.* (1996) Evidence-based general practice: a retrospective study of interventions in one training practice. *BMJ*. **312**: 819–21.

Greenhalgh T (1996) Is my practice evidence-based? *BMJ*. **313**: 957–8.

Hannah R and Greenhalgh T (1997) *A Training Needs Analysis of Primary Health Care Teams in the North Thames Region*. Department of Primary Care and Population Sciences, Whittington Hospital, London.

Kernick D (1997) Which anti-depressant? A commentary from general practice on EBM and health economics. *Br J Gen Prac*. **47**: 95–8.

Kerrison S, Clarke A and Doehr S (1997) *People and Paper – a survey of consultants, GPs and nurses on information sources and information needs for evidence-based medicine in North Thames*. Department of Public Health and Policy, Health Service Research Unit, London School of Hygiene and Tropical Medicine, London.

McColl A, Smith H, White P and Field J (1998) General practitioners' perception of the route to EBM – a questionnaire survey. *BMJ*. **316**: 361–5.

NHSE (1997) *A First Class Service: quality in the New NHS*. Department of Health, London.

NHSE (1999) *The NHS Performance Assessment Framework*. Department of Health, Wetherby.

Rosenberg W and Donald A (1995) Evidence-based medicine as an approach to clinical problem solving. *BMJ*. **310**: 1122–26.

Sackett D, Rosenberg W *et al.* (1996) Evidence-based medicine: what it is and what it isn't. *BMJ*. **312**: 71–2.

Secretary of State (1997) *The New NHS: modern, dependable*. Department of Health, London.

CHAPTER 12

Prescribing: remedy needed for chronic inflation

David Coleman

Good and bad practice are stuck in their own ghettos.[1]

Posing the right questions

Prescribing expenditure, which is now around £4.5 billion annually, is approximately 17% of the primary care budget. In relative terms, then, not by any means the greater part. Nevertheless, it is a major cause for concern because the cost of medicines in primary care has consistently outstripped inflation (averaging over 8% growth year on year for ten years) for almost as long as anybody connected with it can remember. This growth is in spite of huge amounts of sophisticated effort poured into providing information both to support prescribers' decision making, and to inform them about the way they are spending the taxpayer's money. Prescribing expenditure control runs through each of the four litmus tests promoted for effective PCT resource management in Chapter 3.

An obvious retort, and alternative perspective to this central NHS position, is that compared with the rest of the western world, the whole NHS budget is parsimonious to say the least. Therefore, the argument goes, the pressure is almost entirely the result of unrealistic estimates of the real bill for maintaining the nation's health. That there is some truth in this was borne out by the UK Government's pledge in the March 2000 budget to increase NHS expenditure by a third in real terms in five years.

The question of how much of this new money should go on therapeutics is as yet unanswered. It was by no means a high profile inclusion in the popularly labelled 'wish list' published by the Department of Health in the summer of 2000 (Secretary of State 2000). There is a case for some new money to contribute to the cost of new prophylactic initiatives like those in the Coronary Heart Disease National Service Framework and through

---

[1] *NHS Plan* 2000: 2.26

novel initiatives, in cancer care for instance. There is also an argument for reducing what appear to be a small number of interpractice budget inequalities. However, there is no hard evidence overall that the core therapeutic budget should be allowed to grow any more than it has already, and plenty of evidence that it is out of control.

So the big questions for primary care are: is the prescribing budget too big? And how should the current budget be managed? Where do the up and coming pressures for entirely new therapeutics fit in, and should individual GPs continue to have relatively unrestricted access to the public purse to provide for their patients?

Many academics have addressed various issues related to this subject over the last 30 years. In this short chapter, it is impractical to explore the issues in depth. This contribution is the result of the author's observations of some of the issues, made as a community pharmacist of 25 years' standing, a prescribing adviser to various general practices and PCTs, and as a primary care researcher, principally with City and Portsmouth Universities over the 1996–2000 period. Adequate management of existing resources is very important because it is far easier to present a business case for new and expensive therapies against a background of adequate management of the existing budget than in the prevailing climate of repeated failures to contain costs. The story is not merely a matter of cynical cost containment, but rather disinvestment and reinvestment in what is a particularly demanding sphere of management.

Pharmacists' roles in primary care

Pharmacists are now involved in this process at a number of stages. Table 12.1 is an activity analysis which shows where pharmacists currently fit into primary care and their spheres of influence. Their roles are many and various, and undergoing great change. This would have looked quite different five years ago and the change process has further to go, particularly as the authority and powers of primary care trusts (PCTs) develop. Disappointingly, very few were appointed to the boards of PCGs. Will it, I wonder, be different with the new PCT executives?

In the past, the role of the community pharmacist was isolated geographically and politically from most other workers in primary care locations. This is changing slowly, but is hampered as a result of community pharmacists being confined to their pharmacies by their existing legal obligations. One consequence has been that whereas 'top-down' advice to GPs has been accepted in primary care since the mid-1980s, 'bottom-up' initiatives, which are patient-specific and which tend to be, but are not always, community pharmacy driven, are less well established.

Table 12.1   An activity analysis of pharmacists working at various points in primary care

Organisation	Pharmacist appointment	Examples of activities	Principal arena of activity	Main influence
Health authority	• HA pharmaceutical adviser	• Advice on DoH policy, NPC policy, NSF/HImP implications etc. • HA PACT dissemination	• Global policy	• NPC • DoH • DPC
PCG/T	• HA advisers P/T • Freelance advisers • Direct F/T or P/T appointments • P/T community pharmacists	• Similar to above plus direct input into PCG/T prescribing committee, and to prescribing and CG leads • Management of PSPs • EPACT analysis and dissemination		
General practice surgery	• Occasional HA adviser input • Direct FT/PT appointments • Sessional community pharmacists and freelance advisers	• Advice and dissemination of good prescribing practice • Interpretation of PACT reports • Audit • Individual patient prescribing reviews		
Community pharmacy	• Direct appointments and locums • Contracted to proprietor • Proprietors contracted to NHS	• Dispensing prescriptions • Safety scrutiny • Advice on medicine utilisation • Health advice dissemination	• Patient-specific initiatives	• Patients • RPSGB • Medicines Act

NB At PCT level, the HA adviser has no automatic right to see PACT data.
DoH: Department of Health; DPC: District Prescribing Committee; F/T or P/T: Full-time or Part-time; NPC: National Prescribing Centre; PACT: Prescribing Analysis and Costs; PSP: Practice Support Pharmacist; RPSGB: Royal Pharmaceutical Society of Great Britain.

Why is the drug budget so difficult to manage?

I suggest that the single most distinctive reason why it has proved so demanding is that this part of the budget is broken up into a stupendous number of transactions each year (5 million plus in an average health district) with an average value of £8 or £9. This means that a huge number of events, involving dozens of healthcare workers, from the prescriber to the home care worker, need to be effectively co-ordinated. Multi-stage, multi-disciplinary initiatives which are patient-specific and exploit the accessibility of community pharmacists may be the most profitable places to look for the next phase of improvements. Not that this is in any way a denial of the vital importance of the 'top-down' approach. Trust status for PCGs heralds new opportunities to examine these issues. Addressing the following four inter-related priority areas could usefully inform the debate:

- problems which are the result of multiple medication
- medicine concordance – what happens to medication once it is prescribed?
- problems managing repeat medication
- the proposal that PCTs should manage the supply side of their drug budget directly.

A case study: everybody's grandmother

The author has conducted several hundred individual patient medication reviews in the last five years, both as a specific focus of research (Royal Pharmaceutical Society of Great Britain and Merk, Sharpe and Dohme 1997) and in the context of a range of prescribing audits conducted in GP surgeries. The Royal College of Physicians has already pointed to many of the clinical problems created by multiple medication in the elderly, and the following case history presents the issues from a pharmacist's perspective. The case is heavily disguised.

An elderly professional lady, who lives on her own, has diabetes and four other related conditions requiring that she see four different secondary care specialists from time to time. As a result she has a medicine regimen comprising 13 different items and 15 tablets a day, plus insulin injections.

The lady had been known as a careful organiser all her working life, and was now sadly suffering memory loss and confusion as a result of her medical condition. She was visited by the pharmacist as part of a domiciliary visiting programme which was initiated by an audit of chronic pain medicines, applying a methodology based on the pharmaceutical care philosophy of Strand and others (The Royal College of Physicians of London 1997).

She was anxious and concerned because when ordering her medicines she received 'everything she wanted and everything she didn't want'. Unusually, she kept a record of all her daily medication taking in a small diary. The record revealed a level of non-adherence that, though often suspected, is rarely demonstrated so graphically (*see* Box 12.1). It was sufficiently bad to raise serious questions about the value of giving the patient so many medicines.

When asked how she felt on her medicine in the context of administering a structured questionnaire she complained of a maze of difficulties which were the result of side effects, poor medicine adherence, poor understanding of her medicines, and an inability to organise her medicine taking.

Box 12.1   Case study: poor medicine adherence

Number of doses prescribed in 11-day period of analysis	165
Number of doses taken exactly as directed	37
Number of doses taken erratically, i.e. at the wrong time	8
Number of doses doubled up on a given day	2

A questionnaire on beliefs about medicines revealed a patient afraid of addiction and tolerance, inclined to worry that medicines can cause harm, who took her medicines 'according to how she feels'. The patient's notes revealed a history of persistent problems with her diabetes control.

She had boxes and boxes of unwanted medicines stored all over the house. Of particular note were several boxes of insulin. Most were (bizarrely) stored in the bedroom and put in the fridge when she had room, i.e. immediately prior to use (by which time they were probably useless). On examination, the utilisation of insulin revealed it to be relatively modest. The quantity she was receiving was about five times the amount she was taking. The cost of this regimen to the practice was over £3000 per annum. Sorting out the insulin alone reduced this by over £1000.

A report to inform the prescriber included presentation of the issues, including a list of possible and probable adverse reactions as a result of interactions and poor compliance. Recommendations included weekly prescriptions and the supply of her medicines in a unit dose management box (NOMAD) from a local community pharmacy, and a programme of monitoring and support. This lady had been counselled at some length about some of her concerns, but nevertheless needed to be coaxed with considerable sensitivity, over some time, to accept supervision of her medicines in this way. The main obstacle was that it appeared to her to confirm her sense of inadequacy. A programme of rational reduction of doses and prescription items was also embarked upon. This was a joint effort between

prescriber and pharmacist which has started to have demonstrable therapeutic benefits as well as leading to a considerable reduction in prescribing
costs. It was, however, time-consuming, and may continue to be so for
some time.

Although typical in many ways of the difficulties which are encountered
(many readers will have a relative who is elderly who has many of the
problems described) this is a very unusual case because there is clear and
ingenuous evidence that, without close supervision, an expensive (and
elaborate) therapeutic regimen was not having the intended effect. It also
highlights the need to consider who in the continuum from the clinical
specialist in secondary care, through to the pharmacist and the patient, carries the responsibility first for the clinical outcome of therapeutics, and
secondly for managing the drug budget, particularly if something goes
wrong. Where for instance, does the individual patient's freedom of choice
come into the equation? This debate needs to advance on several fronts,
not the least of them being in relation to the pressures on the prescriber to
follow prophylactic medicine protocols, and the ways that prescribing
decisions are devolved from secondary care. Pharmacists' responsibilities
and possible interventions need to be taken into account, particularly with
respect to the management of obviously failing therapeutic outcomes. This
practice would not need to have many patients of this sort to account for
its entire budget overspend.

Fortunately, although perhaps an extreme example, the number of
patients who have this level of need is relatively small. One estimate is that
between 2 and 3% of a practice population have significant unmet pharmaceutical care needs (Cipolle *et al.* 1998). Even at this level, however, the
number might be 4000–6000 patients in a PCT, who are consuming up to
half (i.e. several million pounds' worth) of total drug expenditure. Resolving
these difficulties requires a co-ordinated strategy and minute attention to
detail. It may be an illustration of the great need to move community
pharmacists from a situation in which they are paid for items dispensed to a
more imaginative notion of payment for services. Accordingly, PCTs' local
success in driving better value for money could well lead over time to
major changes in central contractual frameworks for community pharmacists and their staff.

Why don't patients take their medicines? A new way of thinking about prescribing

In North America, evidence emerged in the 1980s and early 1990s that
patients were not conforming to the expectations of the prescribers of
therapeutic regimens. The scale of this appeared to be very significant, with

one research project reporting that adherence might be as low as 50% (Horne 1993). This state of affairs was perceived to be a disaster in social, health outcome and economic terms. In America it has been described as their 'second drug problem'.

In the UK, this was perceived to be so serious an issue that it prompted the production of an expert report in 1997 (Coleman *et al.*). This investigation turned into a huge multi-disciplinary debate on medicine taking to discover 'what is known about the difficulties patients have in taking their medicines as they are prescribed'.

The report concluded that 'research strongly suggests that very many patients are, for one reason or another, unable to take their medicines, this despite prodigious efforts by researchers and practitioners increasingly to make information available to patients and by doctors, pharmacists and nurses to improve their communication skills'. As the issues have become clearer it is evident that precise measurement of medicine adherence is extremely difficult. As a result, the true state of play in the UK remains unconfirmed, although it is recognised as an important issue which needs to be addressed.

The attention of some researchers in the UK has also focused on the reasons for non-adherence, attempting to take further the largely unsuccessful attempts in North America to discover a set of determinants of non-adherent behaviour. It has been demonstrated that the reasons why patients do not take their medicines are very complex and related to the beliefs that they hold about them. Health psychologists have, therefore, often applied social cognition models in an attempt to understand non-adherent behaviour.

Out of the discussion has come the concept of medicine 'concordance' which describes an important cultural shift in the prescriber–patient relationship in which the patient's reactions and beliefs are acknowledged to be a valid contribution to the therapeutic decision. In it:

> The clinical encounter is concerned with two sets of contrasted but equally cogent health beliefs – that of the patient and that of the doctor. The task of the patient is to convey her or his health beliefs to the doctor; and of the doctor to enable this to happen. The task of the doctor or other prescriber is to convey his or her (professionally informed) health beliefs to the patient; and of the patient to entertain these. The intention is to assist the patient to make as informed a choice as possible about the diagnosis and treatment, about benefit and risk and to take a full part in the therapeutic alliance.

Adoption of such a conceptual approach in actual relationships, and the effective dissemination this requires, still constitutes a major cultural challenge for many working in primary care in the UK.

The problem of wasted medicines

The significance of this cultural shift has yet to be widely felt, though pharmacists who regularly see patients find that the conclusions drawn in the report strike a chord with their own experience. Whether or not the patient will take the medicine prescribed is only one of several related problems and I would tentatively propose that a pattern is emerging which begins to explain the ubiquitous problem of wasted medicines. A suggested pathway leading to wasted resources in therapeutics for use by PCTs is described in Figure 12.1.

The burden of large numbers of medicines, difficulties (and perversities) about ordering repeat medicines and the prevention of harm are some of the issues that are widely experienced. Pharmacists in the community probably see the majority of chronic repeat medicine takers more regularly than anyone else in the primary care team. For PCTs they should be ideally placed to manage effective interventions to resolve these difficulties, and indeed are demonstrating in many pilot studies throughout the country (albeit slowly) that they can do so. An imaginative approach to local contracts with community pharmacists is now going to be possible in the context of PCTs and

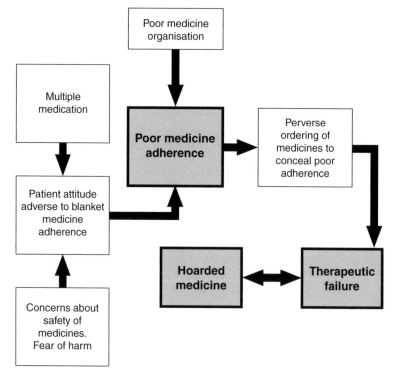

Figure 12.1   A suggested pathway to poor therapeutic outcomes and medicine wastage.

an informed and creative approach could yield a real harvest in years to come. Dorset Health Authority (Coleman) has been pioneering ways of managing a locally devolved contract for pharmaceutical services for many years. This work has been limited in its scope, partly, perhaps, because it was ahead of its time. Numerous pilot studies throughout the country, for instance, are investigating involving community pharmacists in managing repeat prescribing, carrying out domiciliary pharmaceutical care projects and monitoring asthma patients from community pharmacies. A plethora of other opportunities are at various stages of development. There is now much emerging good practice for PCTs to draw upon.

Direct management of the therapeutics budget

If anybody thinks that the problem of prescribing costs begins and ends with purchasing medicines at the lowest price, then I hope that I will have presented enough evidence about the management burden to ask them to think again. Of course, cost containment does require that excessive profits are curbed, but this requires very precise targeting of the culprits, which is an activity which the Department of Health has been engaged in for over 50 years. If, however, multi-disciplinary team working is a key to successful medication management, then one of the axioms on which it will succeed or fail is relational. Harnessing quality relationships between members of the team and the public which they serve is as important to VFM prescribing as recognising that the devil is in the detail.

In an attempt to curb drug prices, propositions which have already been floated by some PCT chief executives include servicing the public directly with, for instance, wound management products, and bringing the community pharmacy 'in house' in some way by making community pharmacists employees of the 'Trust'. This is attractive to PCTs because they are aware of the power of hospital purchasing departments to supply medicines at very deep discounts, and also because there is perceived (with some justification) to be a conflict of interests for community pharmacists paid on an item dispensed basis.

I suggest that these propositions are entertained with some caution and informed by the considerations presented so far which depend upon a co-ordinated effort from (appropriately managed) pharmacists disseminated in the community. There are, however, other considerations which need to be debated thoroughly, as many of the short-term attractions may well turn out to be illusory anyway, in the long run. These include the following.

• The cost of the 'means of production'. The investment in stock alone is about £500 million nationally, let alone the 'goodwill' value of pharmacists, which for most independents represents their pension fund. Also,

PCTs would have to decide if they wish to take over obligations under the Land and Tenancy Act, or leave community pharmacists with an un-supported overhead.

- The attraction of bulk purchasing is based partly on the prices which are achieved by hospital contract purchasers. The difficulty here is that these prices are based on the industry's strategy of selling into secondary care (where the volumes are relatively low) at prices which will establish the product in the market place, and selling into primary care at Drug Tariff prices. In practice, the average price is effectively set by the Prescription Price Regulation Scheme (PPRS), which is subject to constant adjustment, but would effectively ensure that any artificial gains were short lived.

- The attraction of bulk purchasing is further based on the assumption that volume purchasing will secure a large chunk on the wholesaler discount. This also needs thinking through in depth. Most of the medium-sized community pharmacy chains (one of which was once owned by the author) realised in the mid-1990s that the whole market is moving towards a small number of huge vertically integrated companies which wholesale hundreds of millions of pounds' worth of NHS business each. Their steep decline, as they have sold to the large multiples, is testimony in itself to the difficulties which were faced. On the scale of things, individual PCTs tend currently to have drug budgets equivalent just to the small to medium-sized chains which have declined.

Controlling the local activity of community pharmacists (particularly where there are perceived conflicts of interest) may be a better approach than trying to take them over, a strategy which is likely to lead to inheriting all of their problems as well as the advantages. As the most recent central policy guidance suggests (Chief Pharmacist 2000), a better approach might be to consider devising an equivalent model to the Primary Medical Services pilots of the 1997 NHS (Primary Care) Act. There may be scope for PCTs (possibly collectively) to enter the supply chain in the future, although I suspect that most progress would be made in the generics market, and controversially in the market for parallel imported ethicals. Any proposal to radically over-haul the existing commercial system of distribution is at this level likely to face almost as many problems as it addresses. However, control of the contract for pharmaceutical services is an entirely different matter.

Summary

Attempts to control drug expenditure in primary care have historically been an alarming failure. PCTs have therefore inherited responsibility for a major problem. The issues of cost containment and quality of prescribing are inextricably mixed, and pharmaceutical advisers, as well as government advisers, have poured prodigious effort into advising GPs on their decision making, so far with limited success.

Because of their relative isolation, community pharmacists have not been in a position to enter fully into this dialogue, but have been aware from their direct and continuous involvement with the patient, that there are problems which are not really being addressed. However, resolution of these difficulties involves recognition first that the problem exists, and secondly that the time and structures currently in place frustrate addressing the issues in a meaningful way.

Prescribing is characterised by a huge number of events in which dozens of individuals play a part. One of the reasons why it has been so difficult to manage is because recognition of the management challenge is only beginning to emerge as evidence is slowly collected. PCTs will have the power to co-ordinate a multi-disciplinary strategy to bring about change. There is no single quick fix answer, and rather as the search for an answer to the problem of medicine adherence for too long concentrated on the search for easily identifiable non-adherent behaviours and eventually had to give up in the face of the need for a much more complex understanding, so the problem of managing the therapeutic resource will not yield to the writing of protocols and the search for the 'big idea' all on its own. Rather it will be necessary to see that the war is won by mobilising the whole army to move in a co-ordinated way. It will be won by thousands of small changes, effected by a co-ordinated team of people who are motivated to pull together, over time. The relational/team building dimension to achievement in this area is inescapable. The National Prescribing Centre envisages that PCTs will eventually appoint directors of medication management. If the brief is to unify the patient-specific and policy-driven prescribing initiatives in an imaginative way, co-ordinating the entire multi-disciplinary team, this will be a promising initiative. For PCTs, prescribing certainly represents an area of risk, but as both the experience of the NHS and its research evidence show, it is an area where, by comparison with what has gone before, the new trusts can scarcely go wrong.

References

Chief Pharmacist (2000) *Pharmacy in the future: implementing the NHS Plan.* Department of Health, London.

Cipolle RJ, Strand LM, Morley P (1998) *Pharmaceutical Care Practice.* McGraw-Hill, New York.

Coleman DJ (forthcoming publication) *An evaluation of the delivery of pharmaceutical care from a general practice surgery based pharmacy* (PhD Thesis). University of Portsmouth.

Coleman DJ, Portlock J, Brown D (forthcoming publication) *Advancing age and multiple medication as predictors of pharmaceutical care needs.*

Horne R (1993) One to be taken as directed: reflections on non-adherence (non-compliance). *J Soc Admin Pharm.* **10**(4): 150–6.

Royal College of Physicians of London (1997) *Medication for Older People.* Royal College of Physicians, London.

Royal Pharmaceutical Society of Great Britain and Merk, Sharpe and Dohme (1997) *From Compliance to Concordance.* Royal Pharmaceutical Society of Great Britain, London.

Secretary of State for Health (2000) *The NHS Plan.* Department of Health, London.

CHAPTER 13

Practising both care management and managed care

Marie Hill and Roger Hudson

There will be a national framework for partnership between the private and voluntary sector and the NHS.[1]

Context

The White Paper *The New NHS: modern, dependable* (Secretary of State for Health 1997) proposed a radical policy change in the organisation of primary care over the next ten years, with the demise of the controversial NHS internal market to the setting up of primary care groups (PCGs) and trusts (PCTs). These have been delegated specific and challenging responsibilities for:

- addressing health inequalities and ways of improving local health needs
- developing both primary and secondary healthcare services, through investing to improve the quality of care and the integration of services
- commissioning secondary care services.

In order to achieve these objectives, subsequently confirmed in the 2000 *NHS Plan*, PCGs have had to adopt new ways of working, rewriting past pecking orders and creating working relationships based on equity and power sharing with other agencies such as voluntary sector organisations, social care units, patients themselves and the pharmaceutical industry. In so doing they have had to embrace the concepts of both care management and managed care.

---

[1] *NHS Plan* 2000: 11.6

Setting the scene

The National Health Service (NHS) was founded on the principle of providing a health service free to all (regardless of means) at the point of contact, but Aneurin Bevan did not envisage in 1948 that 50 years later the health economy would be so overstretched financially. Ever increasing health demands and advances in medical technology, the increasing aging population, along with more informed and empowered citizens have led to ever-increasing expenditure on the NHS: as a result governments have had to look at ways to ensure that healthcare spending is targeted to appropriate outcomes. So far the analysis is that this has not led to a widespread exclusion of services, but has placed the emphasis on achieving greater cost effectiveness in the use of resources through health technology assessment and evidence-based medicine (Ham 1997).

New ways of delivering information have been developed as alternative ways of providing healthcare in appropriate settings to an ever growing and insatiable population for health promotion. These new initiatives now include the development of NHS Direct, walk-in centres and various triage schemes. In some areas, however, these new developments have not been applauded by the medical profession and have been seen as ways of diluting the power of the general practitioner (GP). PCTs have had to be mindful of the sensitivities of GPs by emphasising that these new initiatives do not replace their key role, but in fact assist this by providing more appropriate services and, therefore, assist the GP in having more time for clinical work. Against this background the Health Improvement Programme (HImP) is designed as a way of addressing local health priorities, seeking to ensure that all residents in specific localities have equal access to comprehensive and cost-effective services. The new alternative sources of health promotion on the one hand and the use of HImPs on the other, to place primary care in a context of clear priorities, indicate how PCG/Ts now need to be both effective practitioners of care management and managed care.

Principles of care management and managed care

Care managers are those with lead responsibilities for organising and arranging care packages for their individual clients. Managed care refers to health or social care schemes at group or collective levels, which provide a defined range of services for a specified population at a set price. Fund-holding was a version of managed care, where clusters of general practices within a district managed resources within a set budget.

With the advent of PCG/Ts there is now a major devolved budget available to them from health authorities to manage the majority of local services. The PCT is both provider and purchaser of services, tailored to meet their specific identified health needs. This tailoring means managed care and the rationing of services is here to stay if PCG/PCTs are to remain within budget.

Making decisions about the allocation of services can, of course, be fraught with ethical dilemmas. This is scarcely an unfamiliar issue and the following are examples of common questions we have encountered in our research and development programmes.

- Who decides what is a just allocation of services from scarce resources?
- Are resources really scarce or are decisions made solely on considerations of staying within budget?
- Does money for a benefit denied to one patient save another patient's life?

In responding to these questions it is PCT Boards that will provide the overall leadership to their respective Executive Committees (ECs). However, it is the EC, as the clinician-dominated board, which is responsible for the operational day-to-day running of the PCT. The EC, therefore, has to demonstrate to the board that its decision making has clear, robust processes. In this role it is strengthened by its new multi-professional character. For example, at least two nurses will be on the EC at both Levels 3 and 4. Nurses and doctors faced with ethical decisions on managed care need to be seen clearly as operating with justice and integrity as advocates for their patients, otherwise patients will distrust the healthcare system. Furthermore, Wurzbach (1998) continues that ethical nursing practice in its implementation requires justice with integrity, that is, treating persons in like circumstances similarly. The advice from the NHS Alliance (Ribchester 2000) suggests a similar requirement for GPs and other primary care professionals, with specialist PCT ethics sub-committees recommended.

Areas of application

Although PCTs can use HImPs to prioritise local health needs, which in turn influence their commissioning decisions, such national priorities as NSFs and winter pressures are 'must dos', regardless of whether these priorities are local priorities. This can place an additional pressure on a PCT to ration remaining services and their expenditure on top of the constraints described in Chapters 3 and 4 in relation to SaFF disciplines. These often restrict PCT flexibilities, at least at first, to the margins of expenditure. In this context integrated care pathways (ICPs) offer a way forward in combining the principles of care management and managed care.

In the UK, pathways are seen as a framework within which to standardise and review the quality of care provided, and to identify and make changes to clinical care, based on the latest evidence and research. An integrated care pathway can help determine and shape locally agreed, multi-disciplinary practice based on guidelines and evidence where available, for a specific patient/client group. It can form all or part of the clinical record, documenting the care given, and can facilitate the evaluation of outcomes for continuous quality improvement. There does need first, however, to be the commitment for change within an organisation to create a culture that is supportive towards integrated care.

Additionally, there needs to be a belief that patients and carers are stakeholders in the care process and the recognition that individual professionals across primary care play an integral part in this process. With these pre-conditions, ICPs are methods of ensuring 'seamless delivery of care'. In PCG/Ts, ICPs are, for example, being introduced through the use of patient handheld notes for multi-disciplinary use, so that information from various professionals flows with the patient and ensures that the duplication of services does not occur. This helps ensure appropriate and cost-effective care, as the following local examples illustrate.

Case study 1

In Newham PCG, Marie Hill undertook project work on developing diabetic patient handheld notes in association with the diabetes specialist nurses. The aim of this work was to ensure that information 'flowed' with the patient, thus avoiding duplication of investigations (i.e. routine glycated haemoglobin (HBA1c, etc.) and that a standardised package of care would be delivered to all diabetic patients. The work was supported by the Diabetes Working Group, which comprised professionals involved in diabetes care. This work has been a valuable exercise and is the basis for proceeding with an ICP framework in diabetes – developed together with the local NHS community trust.

Case study 2

Integrated care pathways take on various forms. The Pathfinder Project, described as 'one stop to health knowledge', was developed by Dr Tom Kennedy at Arrowe Park Hospital Trust. It is a project designed to share health knowledge between clinicians in primary and secondary care. The system is based around clinically useful topics and contains information on:

- when to refer from primary to secondary care
- appropriate investigations
- first line management and service description
- information for patients
- vaccination schedules
- books written by patients and carers to address their own specific areas of interest.

Contribution of external partners

The pharmaceutical industry has worked with primary care for many years. Its utility has been specifically evident in the following areas:

- audit, (e.g. Eli Lilly National Clinical Audit Centre)
- research & development
- training and education initiatives.

These areas are the pillars of managed care and, as the following extended local example indicates, are likely to see PCTs replace practices as the key element in external partnerships with pharmaceutical companies.

Case study 3

Managed care
The County Durham and Darlington Priority Services NHS Trust worked up in 1999–2000 a research project in collaboration with PCG/Ts in County Durham and Darlington SSD and Eli Lilly & Company Limited. The purpose of the project is to assist in the delivery of a comprehensive and high quality responsive mental health service in the County Durham and Darlington localities. It will assist the trusts and their partner agencies in delivering the Mental Health National Service Framework (NSF) agenda and the local County Durham and Darlington Mental Health Strategy, as well as increasing the effective and efficient use of primary care time and resources.

The Mental Health NSF sets clear milestones for developing protocols for the management of schizophrenia between primary and specialist care services by April 2001. It also highlights outcome indicators for severe mental illness. These include monitoring the prevalence of side effects associated with maintenance neuroleptics within a service provider population of people within this client group. The overall aim is to improve the quality of life of service users and their families.

Care pathways

Integrated care pathway development is a pivotal feature of the project. It is currently developing an ICP (product) which enriches the existing interface between primary and secondary care within the Derwentside PCG area, using the Darlington and Dales PCGs as reference groups. The change management process includes implementing the care pathway initially in three pilot sites and eventually across the whole County Durham and Darlington area. It will include early detection and recognition during the pro-dromal phase, adoption of a biopsychosocial model of care, side effect monitoring and engagement improvement. The pathway will be user-centred and evidence-based, and aims to incorporate professional training and development across the relevant stakeholder agencies so as to maximise its effectiveness.

Disease registers

One of the project's objectives is to develop Schizophrenia Disease Registers within the Dales, Darlington and Derwentside PCG areas that span the primary and secondary care interface. This will allow the prevalence of schizophrenia to be established within three pilot sites and promote both the wellbeing of the individual patient and general public safety in allowing resources to be targeted toward those areas with the greatest need. By combining micro- and macroperspective priorities the approach is a classic illustration of future PCT practice in care management and managed care. Registers are a central part of the ICP informing the need for early and effective intervention and promoting protocol usage and implementation.

Ways forward

Health authorities have stringent guidelines on how the NHS can use the resources, facilities and support of the pharmaceutical industry. This has become well incorporated now by the better developed primary care organisations as part of their corporate governance arrangements and is well covered in PCT central guidance (NHSE 1999: Annex A1). In one health authority we have worked with guidelines that stress the use of at least two or more pharmaceutical companies at any one time, so that overt favouritism is not shown to any one company, particularly in the promotion of their products. As Chapter 3 has so powerfully argued, demonstrable probity is the first litmus test of future PCT viability.

Clearly, the pharmaceutical industry has a major role to play within primary care in the future and resources could be provided by this industry where there may be an NHS shortfall of resources to provide certain services. However, professionals, managers and members in the newly emerging

PCTs will, like many health authorities before them, need to ensure that adequate integrity and governance guidelines are in place. Explicit contractual arrangements are essential when entering into any potential working partnership. This has been a basic theme of the private sector and should apply equally in the New NHS (Devlin 1998).

The advent of the PCT and the drive of the HImP to meet locally driven health priorities brings with it ethical dilemmas for its clinicians in balancing finite budgets with the clamour for infinite demands for services within each PCG. Combining care management with managed care as a system driven by clinicians that can balance these demands, offers a way forward through these dilemmas.

References

Devlin M (1998) *Primary Care and the Private Sector*. Radcliffe Medical Press, Oxford.

Ham C (1997) *Health Care Reform – learning from international experience*. Open University Press, Buckingham.

NHS Executive (1999) *Primary Care Trusts: financial framework*. Department of Health, London.

Ribchester J (2000) *Developing Primary Care Organisation Ethics Project Group*. NHS Alliance, Nottingham.

Secretary of State for Health (1997) *The New NHS: modern, dependable*. Department of Health, London.

Wurzbach R (1998) Managed care: moral conflicts for primary health care nurses. *Nurs Outlook*. **46**(2): 62–6.

CHAPTER 14

Realising research can be relevant

Roland Petchey

A new policy on research governance in the NHS will be published.[1]

Research and trust

Hitherto, research has been perceived as a marginal activity for most primary care organisations. The arrival of the NHS PCT brings with it the potential to transform this situation, with unparalleled opportunities for the genuine integration of research into service provision, to the benefit of its patients and the enrichment of the working lives of its providers. We believe that the potential of primary care research extends far beyond its immediate and obvious benefits. It can be an important vehicle for generating trust between provider organisations and the communities they serve, by increasing understanding and reinforcing the commitment to patients and communities and to the whole-person practice that is the hallmark of the best primary care. However, just as PCTs have been struggling to come to terms with their role and function in the New NHS, primary care research (PCR) has also been struggling to develop an identity for itself, after a half-century or more of eking out an existence in the shadow of hospital-based research. As a result, before we can map the way ahead, it is necessary to remind ourselves (if only briefly) of the sometimes rocky road that has been travelled by PCR up to now.

PCR – the past

Historically, reviews of research in primary care have tended to take the form of a litany of the practical barriers to its development (e.g. Chief Scientist's

---

[1] *NHS Plan* 2000: 11.12

Organisation, 1988). This is understandable, because these barriers have been considerable. The first obstacle has been the absence of a *research culture* (or even the presence of a culture that was actively *anti-research*). For one thing, it has been hypothesised that in the past many GPs may have chosen general practice as a means of avoiding involvement in research (much of which appeared to be of dubious value). More fundamentally, it was specu-lated that there might even be a conflict between the culture of general practice (characterised by a pragmatic approach to decision making and a tolerance of uncertainty) and that of research, with its emphasis on abstract knowledge and the reduction (or elimination) of uncertainty (Howie 1998). The second barrier was the absence of *infrastructure support* of the kind that underpinned the activities of researchers in other clinical settings. Would-be primary care researchers had little or no protected time for research, or clerical and technical support for it, or access to the range of specialist research expertise that was taken for granted by their hospital colleagues. The third was lack of opportunities for *research training*. These resource and opportunity constraints were, of course, intensified by the limitations imposed by the organisation of primary care. As long as the independent practice/partnership was the basic organisational building block, few could afford to make the investment needed over the timescales necessary to develop a significant capacity for research and sustain it as an integral prac-tice activity. The result, all too often, was that research remained marginal, supported by the superhuman efforts of a handful of enthusiasts (some-times at considerable personal cost to themselves and their families), and tolerated as an eccentricity (at best) by their colleagues. If their enthusiasm faltered, commitment to research was likely to evaporate.

During the 1990s, a series of policy initiatives has begun to redress this historic imbalance between PCR and acute research. Together, they consti-tute the basic framework of funding and organisation, and PCTs that wish to engage with the research agenda will need to be familiar with it. For example, in 1992, general practice teaching and research won the right to a share of the so-called SIFTR. This is the Service Increment For Teaching and Research which had historically subsidised the teaching and research activities of other clinical academic departments in teaching hospitals (to the tune of £40 000 per medical student at 1990 values). More recently, there has been the development of research practices, initiated by the Royal College of General Practitioners (RCGP) in 1994, and subsequently adopted and extended by the NHS (via 'Culyer NHS Research Funding') (Cox *et al.* 1999). The same period also witnessed the emergence of primary care research networks, such as WReN (Wessex Primary Care Research Network), STaRNet (South Thames Research and Implementation Network) and Trent Focus (Hungin *et al.* 1999). These vary in terms of their origins (some being 'bottom-up' initiatives, while others are more 'top-down') and in their style and structure, but nearly all involve some kind of partnership between an academic centre and practitioners in the field. They all have as their objective that of encouraging primary care workers to develop their own research ideas and to increase their research skills by providing the infrastructure support that had been lacking. Steps have also been taken to create opportunities (such as research training fellowships and joint service–academic appointments) for primary care researchers to undergo systematic education and training in research. Impressive strides have begun to be made, but much remains to be done for PCTs and their partners to recover the deficit.

PCR – towards a definition

Although we have so far concentrated on the practical, financial and organisational barriers to the development of PCR, we have also hinted that there may be more fundamental obstacles to be overcome. Among these is the problem of specifying what we mean by PCR. There are a number of ways we might go about this. One would be to try to define it by its *content*. Thus, an obvious answer might be that it is research into primary healthcare, but this does not help greatly because primary healthcare itself is an extremely elusive concept, that is both historically and culturally variable. In other words, it changes over time as well as from country to country. If we cannot define it by its content, how about trying to define it in terms of its *practitioners* (GPs, practice nurses, nurse practitioners, health visitors, school nurses, social workers, informal carers, etc.)? Or the *sites* where it is practised (the practice, the home, the hospital, the clinic, the school, the nursing home and so on)? Even to try to list the practitioners or the sites of primary care demonstrates the futility of this approach. None of these attempts at definition seems quite adequate. All of them appear to be missing something and they all involve at least a degree of circularity (we have to know what PCR is *before* we can specify who is involved in it or where it is carried out).

Perhaps the central reason that PCR is so difficult to pin down is that, as Howie (1998) has observed, it lacks the theoretical underpinning that is a defining feature of other disciplines. We have already commented on primary care's pragmatism and tolerance of uncertainty. Unlike medicine, which can claim to be based on the biological sciences, as an applied and intensely practical branch of medicine, primary care lacks any obvious uniting theory. It is true that over the years a number of candidates have been proposed. These range from the psychoanalytic theory underpinning the Balint movement in the 1960s and 1970s (Balint 1957) through to insights derived from the social sciences (e.g. Helman 1984; Armstrong

1980) or systems theory (Donabedian 1969). However, none has been capable of providing the sort of comprehensive grand unifying theory (GUT) that has been the Holy Grail of physicists and astronomers over the past two decades. Certainly, none of them has commanded universal assent. If PCR is to realise its potential, however, it is vital that we should be able to place it on some kind of firm theoretical foundation. We believe that the way to achieve this is to take as our point of departure (as before) a specification of what we mean by primary care. This time, however, our purpose is to define it not as a *single* discipline, but as a *cluster of related (but distinct)* disciplines. As we have already seen, the tasks that comprise primary care are extremely varied and diffuse (and becoming ever more so). They encompass medical and social problems, involving illness prevention, health promotion and health education in addition to the treatment of illness. The point we are seeking to make is that these interventions are not only multiple and complex. They also occur at a number of levels, principally spanning individuals, families and communities, but also extending beyond them to include populations, tissues, cells and so forth. These can be arranged into a hierarchy of inclusive systems and sub-systems, as shown in Figure 14.1. However, although this systems framework corresponds closely with the levels at which primary care operates, it is more than that. A moment's thought should reveal that, as we move up (or down) through the hierarchy, we are shifting not just from level to level. We are also shifting between 'ways of seeing' (or theoretical paradigms, if you want to be technical).

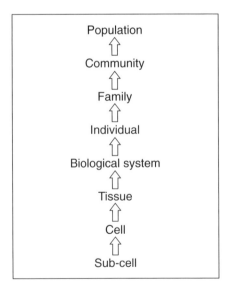

Figure 14.1 PCR – towards a definition.

So, in order to make sense of primary care research, in addition to our hierarchy of systems, we need to introduce two further sets of distinctions. The first of these is our three 'ways of seeing', which we term epidemiological research, health and health service research (H&HSR), and clinical research. The second is the stance which each of these ways of seeing adopts towards the subjective experiences, values and motives of the human subject. Three basic positions can be identified – 'value neutral' versus 'value-laden' versus 'value normative.' (We will define these terms in a moment.) When these are brought together with our hierarchy of systems they produce Figure 14.2.

We should make it clear that the distinctions we are drawing between epidemiology, health and health services research, and clinical research are not intended to represent rigid, watertight divisions. In fact, it is inevitable that there will be considerable overlapping at the boundaries between our three 'ways of seeing'. For example, a clinical researcher whose primary interest is in genetics may well also be interested in the family as a kinship system and in patterns of marriage, since these will affect transmission and

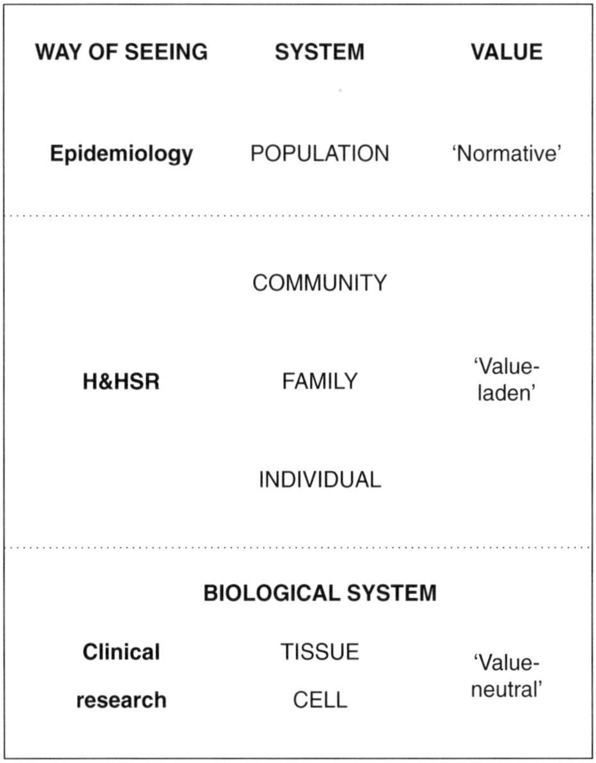

WAY OF SEEING	SYSTEM	VALUE
Epidemiology	POPULATION	'Normative'
	COMMUNITY	
H&HSR	FAMILY	'Value-laden'
	INDIVIDUAL	
	BIOLOGICAL SYSTEM	
Clinical	TISSUE	'Value-neutral'
research	CELL	

Figure 14.2   Hierarchy of research systems.

inheritance. A health services researcher might principally be interested in patients' perceptions of cancer, but might need to have an understanding also of its epidemiology, its aetiology and its staging. The same applies to value neutral, value-laden and value normative: these divisions too will shift up or down the hierarchy of systems, depending on the way of seeing that we are applying. Individually, then, none of these distinctions provides an adequate means of differentiating primary healthcare research from its close neighbours. In combination, however, we believe that they offer PCTs the possibility of identifying some key differences between the various ways of seeing that constitute PCR, with real benefits in terms of discerning relevant research for both application and commissioning as a result. Let us consider each of them in turn.

Epidemiology

Epidemiology is:

> The study of the distribution and determinants of health-related states or events in specified populations, and the application of this study to the control of health problems. (Last 1988: p. 42)

There are a number of features of this definition which merit closer consideration. First, the subject matter of epidemiology is 'health-related states'. Health-related states are not the same as health and illness or disease. They are *abstracted* from the personal, social, cultural and political context in which health and illness are located. This has implications for the way that individuals are conceptualised within epidemiology. It means that they are simultaneously *reduced* to health-related states and *reified* (treated as objects).

The second feature of our definition to note is that epidemiology operates at the level of populations. The *scale* of the population may vary (from the global down through the national to the regional or district or PCT or even practice level). This means that epidemiology is thus quite clearly of considerable potential relevance to PCTs and PCR. However, while the scale of the population may vary, the way it is conceptualised remains constant. For epidemiologists, a population is simply an *aggregation* of individuals who inhabit a given country or area. To exaggerate slightly, epidemiology tends to regard human subjects as disembodied carriers of health-related states or risk factors, or as the medium through which they are distributed. To summarise, epidemiology seems to us to be characterised by *aggregation, abstraction, reductionism* and *reification* of the human subject.

Finally, why have we characterised epidemiology as *value normative*? Tudor Hart (1988: p. 99) provides an answer, drawing attention to what he sees as a fundamental tension between epidemiology's ostensibly apolitical, scientific rhetoric and its inherently (in his view, at least) political nature:

> The language of epidemiology is statistics, a word derived from the same root as the word 'state'. Epidemiology is inescapably a political subject, incapable of social neutrality. The assumptions of epidemiologists about society and its history necessarily and inevitably affect their choice of questions for study, the way they are asked, and the solutions they find credible, however much they conceal this from themselves and their readers by 'value-free' terminology.

In other words, while epidemiology purports to be value-free, it (or much of it at least) implicitly adopts the values that are dominant (or normative) within whichever political framework it happens to be operating.

Clinical research

Although clinical research operates at the opposite end of the systems hierarchy from epidemiology, it has a number of features in common with it. The first is the tendency towards *abstraction*, whereby the condition becomes the object of inquiry rather than the person. Consequently, it too *reifies* and *reduces* its human subjects. The person is reduced to the condition ('the renal failure in Bed 7'). However, in other respects, it differs from epidemiology. Whereas epidemiology aggregates its subjects into populations, clinical research **dis***aggregates* them, by dismantling them (conceptually if not in reality) into biological systems and sub-systems. *Abstraction, reification, reduction* and **dis***aggregation* are defining characteristics of clinical research. Finally, because the individual has been effectively excluded, the clinical researcher is able to adopt a position of *value-neutrality*. Disease states and processes are objective facts. We may sometimes be mistaken about them, or we may not understand them fully (yet), but subjective factors such as values and attitudes are deemed irrelevant to understanding them.

Health and health services research

Epidemiology and clinical research are both likely to be familiar (to some extent) to most of the readers of this book. Successive national 'health of the nation' strategies and recent National Service Frameworks are, in turn, the most obvious examples of each. This is probably not the case with our third 'way of seeing' – health and health services research. For this reason, it seems sensible to spend a little time defining what we mean by it.

If we consider the location of health services research in Figure 14.2, a number of obvious differences should be apparent. The first and most obvious is the level of operation. Where epidemiology aggregates the human subject to the level of the population and clinical research dis-aggregates her/him to the sub-individual biological system level, H&HSR operates at mid-range. Its primary focus is on patients, but conceptualised not as biological systems or as members of a population. Where epidemiology and clinical research reify and reduce the human subject to a clinical condition, or a statistic, H&HSR insists on retaining the human subject at the centre of its enquiry. It regards them as conscious, intending social beings, functioning within a series of inclusive social contexts – families, communities, neighbourhoods and so on.

This brings us to the nub of our argument. We regard H&HSR as important because we see important parallels between its character and the character of primary healthcare itself, which is committed (or at any rate is supposed to be committed) to holistic practice. Both insist on the necessity of embodying the condition in the whole person, in the sense of an individual with a history (by which we mean a personal biography as well as a clinical history), which supplies social meaning and significance to the experience of illness and treatment. Both require that the patient's perception of the condition should be understood and addressed at the same time that any disease is treated. At the same time, both also acknowledge the necessity of locating the patient in the context of a network of relationships consisting of family and community and a system of wider economic, social, cultural and political structures. On the other side of the patient–provider relationship, both also insist on locating the provider in the context of a similar system of economic, social, cultural and political structures and practices. As a consequence, both insist on retaining the full complexity of the interactions between environment, illness, patient and carer as a focus for inquiry.

By doing so, H&HSR accepts the inevitability that values and subjective meanings will be brought to the clinical relationship from both sides. It also accepts the possibility that they may conflict. As a result it is, inevitably and inescapably, *value-laden*.

PCR and PCTs

Simply by virtue of their size, the resources at their disposal and the economies of scale they make possible, PCTs have the potential to transform PCR from an activity that is marginal to primary care to one that is at its core. Released from the constraints of the practice/partnership, for the first time, primary care researchers should be able to look forward to consistent

access to the kind of support and opportunities that hospital-based researchers have taken for granted in the past. Not only do PCTs have the
means to do this, we believe that they should also have the motivation.
The public health and service planning functions that PCTs are responsible
for will mean that epidemiological research is bound to feature prominently
on the PCR agenda, as a tool for understanding local patterns of health and
illness and their determinants. At the same time, PCTs also offer increased
scope for involvement in clinical research, by virtue of the greater patient
numbers which they are capable of delivering to the researcher.

It should be clear that we have no wish to denigrate the potential useful-
ness of epidemiology and clinical research to PCTs, but rather our aim is to
help ensure that they are applied neither inappropriately nor exclusively
to such new complex developments in primary care as the waves of PMS
pilots which require an alternative more rounded approach. Both of them
are clearly important tools to PCTs in discharging their responsibilities for
planning services and measuring their effectiveness. In both of them PCTs
also enjoy advantages, which were not available to stand-alone practices.
However, we believe that there is a special and particular affinity between
H&HSR and primary care, in terms of the shared values and perspectives
that underlie the two. We want to argue that this vision of PCR confers on
PCTs a number of significant advantages. The first (and most obvious) is
the opportunity to pursue a research agenda which is shaped by PCTs' own
needs and concerns (rather than by, for example, the priorities of drug
companies or clinical researchers). For instance, many PCTs are faced with
the task of extending services to patient groups who have historically
been either excluded from traditional general practice/primary care or else
under-served by it. This will mean that PCTs will need not only to look
outward to investigate and understand the values and behaviours of *patients*,
they also to look inward to scrutinise *their own* values and behaviours as
providers. To give just one example, our research with people with HIV/
AIDS found a systematic mismatch between their expectations and experiences regarding the maintenance of confidentiality and those of the practice
staff with whom they interacted (Petchey, Farnsworth and Williams 2000;
Petchey, Farnsworth and Heron, forthcoming).

If we are to understand their concerns (and those of people like them),
we have to see them in context. This means seeing them as rational and
reasonable responses to their condition and their attempts to manage it.
From this first, indispensable step in the change process we can then go on
to review patterns of provision and organisation, with the aim of making
them more accessible and acceptable. It is because this style of research
almost inevitably involves those considerations that we earlier suggested
that it could serve as a vehicle for PCTs in engendering trust and building
relationships with the community.

Suggestions for further reading

Carter Y and Thomas C (eds) (1999) *Research Opportunities in Primary Care*. Radcliffe Medical Press, Oxford. This book provides a comprehensive introduction to, and overview of, a wide range of opportunities for research in primary care. Although it pre-dates the advent of PCG/Ts, it is probably the most up-to-date guide available.

Bowling A (1997) *Research Methods in Health*. Open University Press, Buckingham. A comprehensive, authoritative and (crucially) accessible introduction to just about every research method you are ever likely to need, by one of the leading health researchers.

References

Armstrong D (1980) *An Outline of Sociology as Applied to Medicine*. John Wright & Sons, Bristol.

Balint M (1957) *The Doctor, his Patient and the Illness*. Pitman, London.

Chief Scientist's Organisation (1988) *Report of the Working Group on Research in Health Care in the Community*. Chief Scientist's Organisation, Edinburgh.

Cox J, Farmer A and Seamark D (1999) Research practices. In: Y Carter and C Thomas (eds) *Research Opportunities in Primary Care*. Radcliffe Medical Press, Oxford.

Donabedian A (1969) *A Guide to Medical Care Administration. ii Medical care appraisal quality and utilization*. Health Administration Press, Ann Arbor.

Helman C (1984) *Culture, Health and Illness*. Wright, London.

Howie, J (1998) Research in general practice. In: I Loudon, J Horder and C Webster (eds) *General Practice under the National Health Service*. Oxford University Press, Oxford.

Hungin P, Kendrick T, Moore M *et al.* (1999) Research networks. In: Y Carter and C Thomas (eds) *Research Opportunities in Primary Care*. Radcliffe Medical Press, Oxford.

Last J (1988) *A Dictionary of Epidemiology*. Oxford University Press, Oxford.

Petchey R, Farnsworth B and Heron T (forthcoming) The maintenance of confidentiality in primary care: a survey of policies and procedures. In: *AIDS Care*.

Petchey R, Farnsworth B and Williams J (2000) 'The last resort would be to go to the GP.' Understanding the perceptions and use of general practitioner services among people with HIV/AIDS. *Soc Sci Med*. **50**: 233–45.

Tudor Hart J (1988) *A New Kind of Doctor*. Merlin Press, London.

PART 3

Looking ahead

Derek Cramp, Geoff Meads and Fedelma Winkler

CHAPTER 15

Regaining public confidence

The NHS must be re-designed to be patient centred.[1]

Achievement and aspiration

> Never go on a platform to speak about what you plan to do.
> Only speak about what you have done.

This was wise counsel, from an experienced and respected health authority chief executive whose district had, and still has, an outstanding track record. It is achievements not aspirations that really matter. Believe in behaviour not words alone, which too easily become boasts. These principles are apposite for the contemporary NHS where, as we have seen in the preceding chapters, realising a reciprocal and productive relationship between central policy and local practice is a constant and ever more demanding challenge.

Looking ahead, where does the July 2000 *NHS Plan* (Secretary of State 2000) fit into this context? Does its operational focus represent a pragmatic recognition of the dilemma facing a government seeking to both enhance decentralisation and direction? Or do the bold, long-term targets which, on examination, sometimes simply seem to be present trends accentuated, fall into the category of aspirations based more on style than substance? Is the plan to be trusted? To repeat the thematic of this book, set out in its first chapter, will the future PCTs, and their successors, live up to their name with all the meanings each term in their title implies?

In the past, as Chapter 16 demonstrates, the ethical integrity of the NHS has depended upon its professions. Their ethical principles and foundations have been implicitly accepted throughout the history of the NHS as the guarantors of what the new NHS plan describes as 'a health service designed around the patient' (Executive Summary: p. 1). The patient's wellbeing was understood to automatically come first. Now it is understood that it did not, or at least in reality, not enough. By themselves, professional safeguards

---

[1] *NHS Plan* 2000: 1.3

alone are regarded as no longer satisfactory. In the same plan the Secretary of State himself asserts:

> The problem for today's NHS is that it is not sufficiently designed around the convenience and concerns of the patient. The NHS provides many patients with a good and reliable service. But it is simply not responsive enough to their needs. (Introduction: pp. 1–2)

The professions are seen now as part of the problem with their 'old fashioned demarcations' (Introduction: p. 2), 'unnecessary boundaries' (2.18), 'absence of clear national standards' (2.15) and, above all, terms and conditions which remain 'too much the product of the era in which it was born' (2.10), producing a 'relationship between service and patient [which] is too hierarchical' (2.33). They are too, of course, to be fair also fully recognised as part of the solution:

> Clinicians and managers want the freedom to run local services. They want to be able to shape services around patients' needs. (2.32)

But, as the above indicates, they are not the sole solution. Healthcare will be managed, and it will be managed to centrally determined policies and priorities. It is on politicians not professions, now, in the last analysis, that the 'patient-centred' NHS should rely. This clearly is the modern message.

Future scenarios

The primacy of individual relationships has given way to those at organisational or even multi-organisational levels. The heroic tradition of the omni-competent, 24-hours-a-day general practitioner upon which fundholding was founded appears to be coming to an end. By contrast, national political leadership of the health and healthcare system is being revived, albeit in novel regulatory guises, as the UK national government asserts its future identity in terms of those themes which transcend the roles and responsibilities that can be devolved to regional assemblies, unitary authorities and elected mayors. Unequivocally, along with defence, prosperity, Europe, education and security, health and healthcare are among these. And with these changes the conventional divide between the public and private sectors implodes. As a consequence, simple, hierarchic formal organisational structures are becoming redundant, as the state of the United

Kingdom, through its political leadership, looks to legitimately shape relationship processes in pursuit of desired outputs and outcomes, regardless of their location.

Looking ahead for PCTs, this shift from ultimate professional to political accountability offers a range of scenarios, each of which is equally tenable. Politics, after all, is a continuous change process. The average tenure of a modern Secretary of State for Health is two years. For several Ministers of Health their role has served as pre-Treasury experience in a major service department and a career stepping-stone. Governments last five years at a time and often only five years, depending on General Election results. Political values and their emphasis differ over time with these changes. PCTs could just as easily in the future be the springboard for competitive tendering as they are now for combining health and social services frontline personnel. Many types of proprietorship are potentially on offer. They are already, after all, companies which require, by law, only majority NHS funding. They could signal the conversion of general practices into a nationalised set of service outlets – the end of the GP as we have known him/her – or the conversion of the NHS itself into a massive network of small healthcare businesses. It is a time for anti-heroes.

Anti-heroes

The power afforded GP fundholding, with its emphasis on local diversity and the pre-eminence of the sovereign general medical practice in the primary care-led NHS, helped create further space for the entrepreneurs in general practice to develop organisations and services designed to deliver optimum care for their patients. Unquestionably these GPs have been, and have been presented and perceived as *the* heroes of primary healthcare. With the advent of PCTs this position has to be questioned, and questioned from the perspective of the overall public interest. To whose benefit should PCTs' decisions be directed?

Can they, or should they continue to build entire systems of healthcare on the outlier? An edifice built on the right of the curve is in danger of toppling over the rest. Recent declines in GP morale and recruitment suggest that in the 1990s this has become an increased danger. For the public, at the same time, individual GPs have been placed at the pivotal points of changing structures with additional responsibilities for commissioning and services in the community. With those changes the GP has become the principal co-ordinator for the care of the individual. But the doctrines of professional autonomy and local diversity, allied to a monopoly status as the exclusive and independent contractors for general practice, means that until the turn of the century there have been no protective mechanisms for the patient whose GP chooses not to care.

To address this fundamental flaw, PCTs will need to become poachers turned gamekeepers, as was frequently argued by those preparing the ground for the new NHS reforms. The doctrine of local diversity has invariably reinforced the inverse care law (Winkler 1996; Audit Commission 1996). Enforcing the variations in general practice has benefited the patients of entrepreneurial practices in affluent areas. Historically, changes in general practice have been built upon assumptions that the rising tide would lift all. Every GP would be swept along on the waves of best practice. PCTs must re-examine this proposition.

In applying 'who benefits?' criteria this shall inevitably mean that future requirements of maintaining public confidence and sustaining the local credibility of a national health service with its patient customers will cause PCTs to revisit the independent status of practitioners. Optimum primary care and primary care-led commissioning can no longer be left to the vicissitudes of small businesses. They have to be developed within a clear strategic framework and a modernised structure that go beyond general practice to the public guarantee of holistic services in primary care.

General practice has been part of an independent small business sector which, in modern times, is contracting and changing towards high quality, high cost and specialist outlets. The non-specialists are increasingly being driven out of business, unless they adopt different organisational structures. For general practice a useful analogy for the purposes of transferable learning is farming. Farmers too are usually small businesses, peculiarly susceptible to financial incentives, and dependent on public subsidy. Again, as with general practice, the reward system historically has penalised the developers in farming and protected the weaker, and it is only recently, under the influence of European legislation, that the inefficient have been taken over by the better performers.

In general practices the same stresses are present as in any small business. The high quality outlets have developed and the New NHS will ensure that they are increasingly visible. The legal partnership format clearly restricts their future service and economic potential, and the public, it may be assumed, are on their side. The role of PCTs will be to convert the potential into the public interest. This is, in effect, their franchise as a new organisation.

The franchise method of combining equity and access is, after all, already well established with the public in a franchise system. Each outlet remains independently owned but must adhere to quality and service standards. The owners trade freedom to operate their business in individual ways for the right to offer branded services. They benefit from the pooled resources. The risks and rewards are shared. Scope for expansion is available by increasing customers on one site; by increasing the numbers of sites, or by becoming the lead franchise responsible for the performance of other service outlets. All three routes are possible for PCTs to take, depending on their different circumstances.

The franchise system is a modern organisational structure made for PCTs. In the commercial sector, the likes of Virgin have helped ensure that it has gained the public's confidence. In the voluntary sector, Citizens' Advice Bureaux operate to a classic franchise model and are again held in high public esteem. For the professional classes in PCTs, perhaps the most attractive element to the franchise system is that it provides a framework for genuine accountability without excessive standardisation. Conformity is, after all, for better or worse, still anti-cultural in UK primary care.

Collaboration

No system, of course, is without its pitfalls. A deep commitment to the community, a public service ethos and a culture of collaboration need to be part of PCTs if they are to enable the public to regain confidence in the NHS. These qualities need to be reinforced in the PCT franchises' formal terms and conditions.

Back in 1972, legislation in Finland successfully sought to shift the emphasis towards the development of preventive and open care. The new Primary Health Care Act then directed a much higher proportion of new resources than hitherto to primary care development, with a supportive financial and administrative infrastructure that has since ensured priority for geographically and socially marginal areas. In New Zealand's new community organisations and many Health Care Co-ops in the USA, user involvement in decision making is built in at every stage of the care cycles, starting with the primary care clinic. In parts of the Netherlands it is older people themselves through their own local councils who take the ultimate responsibility for steering their primary and community care service developments. In terms of the scale of participation described in Figure 15.1 they are clearly near the top end. In this country we have usually experienced the NHS from the bottom rungs.

But it is possible to climb the ladder; if you are fit and brave enough. For PCTs this strength and confidence now depends upon collaboration. If internally the professionals can learn to be inter-professional then this can be the basis and prerequisite for external collaboration with patients and the public. This is why PCTs can be regarded as one of the participatory elements in the renewal of democracy. Collaboration between primary care professionals is part of modern societies' attempts, globally, to involve patients in decision making. But unless the people delivering the services feel involved, they will not be able to involve their patients and community.

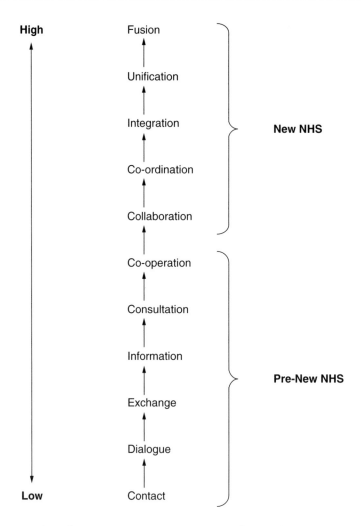

Figure 15.1 Scales of participation. *Source*: HMG teaching aid 1998–2000

Collaboration is often justified on the grounds of individual psychological benefit, as an interpersonal value, or even on economic and financial grounds as a pathway to efficient skills substitutions. In the UK, indeed, the contemporary debate is now almost exclusively concerned with the delivery of cost-effective care. The policy is to develop nursing skills to take on work previously undertaken by doctors, of whom, by European standards, there continues to be a numerical shortfall. Nevertheless, this trend is still threatening to doctors. Subsets of both medical and nursing leadership oppose the direction of travel. There is little research literature to back up the policy, which, as a result, often seems to be among the least explicit and visible of central initiative.

Nevertheless, in terms of espoused behaviour it is a real policy emerging from the expressed statements of the *New NHS*. Its ultimate justification is the popularity of nurses. They do possess the confidence of patients and the public. PCTs need to recognise these realities. As national frameworks, education commissioning structures, research regimes and institutional arrangements adjust over the next decade to both a multi- and interprofessional focus, the new PCTs will have to become wedded to a culture of collaboration. For them the realities of securing public confidence are that the benefits of being seen to work together go beyond simply the social and economic. Their legitimacy as organisations in their patients' eyes will depend upon it.

The way ahead

To approach the options described in this chapter and to make sense of them it is now, finally, important for PCTs to apply scenario planning with the same rigour as the strategic approach adopted for the NHS plan. Unlike the latter, scenario planning operates to complex theory rules: minor adjustments to modern systems may cause major impacts; these adjustments are often unpredicted and unexpected; but clustering variables and defining trends does, nevertheless, allow a degree of confidence in suggesting what the determinants of tomorrow's organisational developments, especially in primary care, might be (Griffiths and Byrne 1998).

It is with this approach in mind that the following closing chapter addresses the future scenarios for PCTs. In this, Derek Cramp guides us in elegantly distilling the learning from the individual contributors to this book and offers a framework to help PCTs approach the difficult decisions they must now make with integrity. Restoring an ethical basis to healthcare is probably just about the biggest contribution that PCTs can make to the NHS, its patients, its professionals, and, in particular, its politicians.

References

Audit Commission (1996) *What the Doctor Ordered: a study of GP fundholders in England and Wales*. HMSO, London.x

Griffiths F and Byrne D (1998) General practice and the new science emerging from the theories of 'chaos' and complexity. *Br J Gen Pract*. **48**: 1697–9.

Secretary of State (2000) *NHS Plan*. Department of Health, London.

Winkler F (1996) Collective and individual responsibilities. *Prim Care Management*. **6**(7/8): 2–8.

CHAPTER 16

Taken on trust: an essay on reflective decision thinking[1]

Trust is still the glue that binds the NHS together.[2]

Did you ever expect a corporation to have a conscience, when it has no soul to be damned and no body to be kicked. (Attributed to Lord Chief Justice Thurlow; 1778–92)

Introduction

This chapter is by way of being an essay in what I call reflective decision thinking, a phrase that might be regarded as synonymous with ethical decision making. But why might this be thought to be an appropriate way of rounding off, in a somewhat philosophical manner, the excellent chapters that have gone before? As one reads these chapters it is impossible not to be impressed with the organisational complexity of modern primary care, the difficulties that must inevitably arise in its management and especially in the decision-making process. An obvious example is deciding on the efficient allocation of resources, where all too often demand exceeds supply and thus involves the creation of some order of priorities. It requires choosing appropriate issues for attention, setting objectives, considering feasible alternative courses of action and making choices from these alternatives. Fixing agendas, setting objectives and determining possible actions is conventionally called problem solving, while evaluating and making choices is called decision making.

As PCT board and EC members are now discovering, decision makers are interested in making good decisions, or, more precisely, making decisions that have good outcomes. But, as March (1982) succinctly puts it: 'actual

---

[1] We wish to thank Helen Winter for her constructive comments on this paper.
[2] *NHS Plan* 2000: 1.2

decision making, particularly in organisations, often contrasts with the vision of decision making implicit in theories of choice'. In the real world, planning for policy implementation involves so many factors, concerns and activities that it becomes very difficult for decision makers to give all of them balanced consideration. Inevitably, there is a tendency to 'muddle through' (Lindblom 1959) with subjective judgements rather than objective evaluations all too often determining choice.

The heroic days of general practice that existed up until the 1960s, as chronicled for instance in the novels of AJ Cronin and the factual accounts of such practitioners as Julian Tudor Hart (1988), are long gone. Managed care is now the main background to the primary healthcare enterprise, driven by a perceived need to contain healthcare costs by making health-care interventions more efficient through evidence-based clinical practice and improved decision making. After all, if there is a range of acceptable options why not go for the least expensive and why not treat only those most likely to benefit from treatment? The new thinking may produce better population care and almost certainly makes for better economics, but what scope does it provide for meeting the needs of people and supporting them when they are at their most vulnerable? Indeed, to what degree can an organisation be a 'caring organisation' when present policy is directed towards greater centralisation and control, and, in spite of the avowed inten-tions, making the concept of local management a fiction and, in fact, reviving the concept of efficient administration?

In a way, this is the culmination of a process that started some 50 years ago when ideas and criteria for improving the efficiency and quality of healthcare delivery were introduced from commerce and industry. It tends to be forgotten that the structure-process-outcome model associated with the name of Donabedian, the diagnostic related group model developed at Yale by Fetter and colleagues, the TQM movement and business process re-engineering, all had a direct industrial or commercial provenance. The net result is that all too often, despite the sophistication of approach, reduc-tionist, simplifying assumptions lead to 'simplistic thinking'. That para-doxically results in 'complex solutions' such as target numbers, league tables, etc. But this is the world we are in, the world of the third way.

It seems to be forgotten sometimes that our organisational resources are there to help people regain health, avoid illness or to live with infirmity or chronic disease as well as possible. But there is another dimension and this is that in the caring process the personal values of those being helped will be taken into account. Indeed, Kass (1985) maintains medicine, and thus by extrapolation I suggest healthcare, is a 'moral enterprise'. Thus if values are intrinsic to decisions the 'ought' or ethical dimension should be an integral part of thinking about how healthcare is delivered. This is the realm of ethics.

What is ethics?

Ethics is concerned with values and behavioural relationships between persons, with norms of right and wrong, of what is thought to be good or bad, of 'ought' and 'ought not'. Values are at the heart of ethics; they govern how we treat each other and the systems we create to bring about the care of one another. Ethical decision making involves ethical reasoning and behaviour about best action, based on the conviction that some actions are better than others. Moral and ethical thinking explores relationships between people about how to live well as a human community. Ethical issues permeate an enormous spectrum of healthcare practice, from the way we greet other people to making a decision to stop a particular intervention or course of action; from the way research is conducted to the way we relate to other professionals in the healthcare team (Downie and Calnan 1994).

Some ethical concerns

Ethical issues for healthcare professionals may be recognised in several guises, as:

- ethical violations that occur as the result of incompetence, carelessness, or deliberate wrong-doing
- ethical dilemmas that arise as a result of the tension that can exist when two or more alternative courses of action of equal moral worth are available
- ethical distress generated by feelings of guilt, concern or distaste arising from an awareness of inappropriate actions or inactions imposed on a person in care.

It will be immediately recognised that such ethical concerns originate in the context of our attitudes to others and our perceived relationships with them and the quality of the decisions thinking made in healthcare situations.

The nature of ethical thinking is to consider appropriate action by asking such questions as the following.

- What are the obvious or hidden values that influence action?
- Whose and what values are given priority?
- What are the diverse opinions influenced by societal norms, by religious perspectives, or by different cultural perspectives?
- What principles guide actions?
- How do we care for one another?

Relationships

As these questions are considered by PCTs and the other responsible players in the New NHS the whole arena of human relationships has to be addressed, for relationships are at the centre of ethical discussion and debate. In healthcare, ethics has to do with relationships between healthcare providers and patients, between healthcare disciplines, between employers and employees, and between government and communities. Relationships are at the centre of questions like:

- what are the values, beliefs and wishes of the patient/client?
- what are the values, beliefs and wishes of the healthcare professional?

There are several different types of relationship in healthcare, based upon patterns of authority and responsibility. These relationships represent a continuum in the types of relationships possible, depending on the degree of responsibility and accountability. Several models of relationship have been formulated and described, and two of these, the fiduciary model and the partnership model, are particularly relevant to our discussion in the context of PCT development.

The fiduciary partnership

There is increasing societal value placed on human rights, including rights to information and rights to personal decision making about one's body and about healthcare interventions. In this context, a partnership model with greater equality in the professional–client relationship is broadly accepted as the model for good healthcare. A relational ethic accepts that both patients and professionals are individuals with beliefs and values that may differ. This ethic also accepts that individuals act on their own behalf. It involves partners who are sensitive to the particulars of the situation, with respect and attention to notions of choice, tact, and emotion. But it should be noted that a relational ethic is a process, not an outcome.

Context

A relational ethic always occurs within a context that includes several levels of relationship – society, institution and family as well as the individual. Each context provides important detail about ethical situations for every participant, usually from a variety of unique perspectives. The societal context of healthcare and ethics tends to be dominated by medical technology, with an emphasis upon, and a preference for, quantitative data with less attention being paid to the importance of people and human relationships. This preference affects the way we evaluate or assess human needs, encouraging an approach to ethical decision making rather like a problem-solving exercise. This approach may often minimise the context of the web of important relationships unique to each situation.

Society, equity and economics

As a result of the managed care approach a high value is placed on efficiency and cost-cutting measures. Inevitably, this presents a challenge to values, to the principle of equity and the criteria of universality, comprehensiveness and accessibility. Such concerns are becoming reflected in a political shift in values and beliefs that in turn are producing changes in personal values and beliefs.

Values and beliefs

A value such as trust is defined as that which is desirable or esteemed for its own sake, something that is prized, cherished, or regarded as highly important. When values are placed in the context of moral values, these values generate rights and duties. A belief is the conviction that something is true. Within the partnership model, there is recognition that values and beliefs are both shared and individual. Partners in relationship each have the ability and responsibility to act within a personal value system. While there are legal and ethical values held communally, individuals (both patients and professionals) have beliefs that must be respected and held to account in partnership relationships. As with context, several layers of values inform the ethical questions and actions in their practice. Some ethical values have gradually evolved into legal principles.

The four ethical principles

Another way to express values is through the development of principles derived from ethical theory (Beauchamp and Childress 1994). Interpretations of principles vary, and our understanding of their application to practice continues to evolve. Principles do not provide a template for action. In the realm of healthcare it is difficult to hold rules or principles that are absolute. This is due to the many variables that exist in the context of clinical cases as well as the fact that in healthcare there are several principles that seem to apply to many situations. Even though they are not considered absolute, these rules and principles serve as powerful action guides in clinical medicine and are perceived by many to be helpful in the moral analysis of ethical issues in medicine. Principles assist in ethical decision making regarding ethical action in a particular situation.

How do principles 'apply' to a particular situation?

Some ethical principles of healthcare appear to have self-evident value, for example:

- the notion that the clinician 'ought not to harm' any patient (*primum non nocere*) appears to be convincing to any rational person
- the idea that the clinician should develop a care plan designed to provide the most 'benefit' to the patient in terms of other competing alternatives also seems self-evident
- it is commonly accepted that before commencing a course of treatment a patient must indicate a willingness to accept the proposed treatment, if the patient is mentally competent to do so
- medical benefits should be dispensed equitably and those with similar needs and in similar circumstances will be treated with fairness.

It might be argued that all these principles should be taken into account if they are applicable to a particular clinical case. Yet, when two or more principles apply they may be found to conflict. For example, a patient with acute abdominal pain is diagnosed to have appendicitis; the medical goal would be to provide the greatest benefit by operating. But, surgery and general anaesthesia carry some small degree of risk to an otherwise healthy patient, and we are under an obligation 'not to harm' the patient. However, a rational calculus suggests that the patient is in far greater danger from harm from a ruptured appendix than from the surgical procedure and anaesthesia. In other words, there is a *prima facie* duty both to benefit the patient and to 'avoid harming' the patient. However, in real life, the demands of these principles must be balanced by determining which carries more weight in the particular case. *Prima facie* duties are always binding unless they are in conflict with stronger or more stringent duties. A moral person's *actual* duty is determined by weighing and balancing all competing *prima facie* duties in any particular case.

What are the major principles of healthcare ethics?

The commonly accepted principles of healthcare ethics include:

* respect for autonomy
* non-maleficence
* beneficence
* justice.

Respect for autonomy (recognising the capacity of an individual to decide what should be done to their body). Any notion of moral decision making assumes that rational agents are involved in making informed and voluntary decisions. In healthcare decisions, respect for the autonomy of the patient would, in common parlance, mean that the patient has the capacity to act intentionally, with understanding and without any influence being brought to bear that would mitigate against or hinder a free and voluntary act. This principle is the basis for the practice of 'informed consent' in the physician–patient transaction regarding healthcare.

The principle of non-maleficence (doing no harm to the patient). The principle of non-maleficence requires that no needless harm or injury is caused to a patient, either through acts of commission or omission. In common language, it is considered to be negligent if a careless or unreasonable risk of harm is imposed upon another. Providing a proper standard of care that avoids or minimises risk of harm is supported not only by commonly held moral convictions, but by the laws of society as well. In a professional model of care one may be morally and legally blameworthy if one fails to meet the standards of due care. In general terms legal criteria for determining *negligence* are as follows:

* the professional must have a duty to the affected party
* the professional must breach that duty
* the affected party must experience a harm and
* the harm must be caused by the breach of duty.

This principle affirms the need for medical competence. It is clear that medical mistakes may occur; however, this principle articulates a fundamental commitment on the part of healthcare professionals to protect their patients from harm.

There is a category of cases that is confusing since a single action may have two effects, one that is considered a good effect, the other a bad effect. How does a duty to the principle of non-maleficence direct us in such cases? The formal name for the principle governing this category of cases is usually called the *principle of double effect*. A typical example might be the question as to how to best treat a pregnant woman newly diagnosed with carcinoma of the uterus. The usual treatment, removal of the uterus is considered a life-saving treatment. However, this procedure would result in the death of the fetus. What action is morally allowable, or, what is our duty? It is argued in this case that the woman has the right to self-defence, and the action of the hysterectomy is aimed at preserving her life. The unintended consequence (though undesired) is the death of the fetus. There are four conditions that usually apply to the principle of double effect:

- the action itself must not be intrinsically wrong, it must be a good or neutral act
- only the good effect must be intended, not the bad, even though it is foreseen
- the bad effect must not be the means of the good effect
- the good effect must outweigh any morally dubious effects and is permitted.

Other problems arise when the patient cannot decide for himself and others must determine what is in the best interest of the patient, or what constitutes the lesser harm.

The principle of beneficence (literally acting in the patient's best interest). The ordinary meaning of this principle is the duty of healthcare providers to be of benefit to the patient, as well as to take positive steps to prevent and to remove harm from the patient. These duties are viewed as self-evident and are widely accepted as the proper goals of medicine. These goals are applied both to individual patients, and to the good of society as a whole. For example, the good health of a particular patient is an appropriate goal of medicine, and the prevention of disease through research and the employment of vaccines is the same goal expanded to the population at large. It is sometimes held that non-maleficence is a constant duty, that is, one ought never to harm another individual, whereas beneficence is a limited duty. A physician has a duty to seek benefit for all of his patients. However, the GP may also choose who to admit onto his practice list, and does not have a strict duty to benefit patients not on his list. This duty becomes complex if two persons seek treatment at the same moment. Some criteria of urgency of need might be used, or some principle of first come first served, to decide who should be helped at the moment.

The principle of justice is the allocation of scarce medical resources between different groups and between individual patients in a fair or equitable manner. Justice in healthcare is usually defined as a form of fairness, or as Aristotle once said, 'giving to each that which is his due'. This implies the fair distribution of goods in society and requires that we look at the role of entitlement. The question of distributive justice also seems to hinge on the fact that some goods and services are in short supply, there is not enough to go around, thus some fair means of allocating scarce resources must be determined. Rawls (1972) claims, and many others agree, that many inequalities are a result of a 'lottery' for which the affected individual is not to blame, therefore, society ought to help by providing resources to help support the disadvantaged. It is a hallmark of the NHS that it attempts to be beneficent and fair and provide a minimum level of healthcare for all, regardless of ability to pay.

Resource allocation

Often it is difficult, if not impossible, to provide every patient with every-thing necessary to provide optimal medical care. So, in conditions of scar-city it may be necessary for PCTs to make trade-offs in some way and allocate resources in a fair and compassionate manner.

What rules guide rationing decisions?

Rationing occurs when many people are in need of an intervention but for some reason that intervention is in short supply. The reasons vary: there are many more patients with end-stage renal disease than there are organs available for transplant; expensive equipment may be lacking; tertiary care hospital beds may be limited; a particular drug may be extremely costly.

The allocation of organs for transplant is highly organised and criteria exist for matching available organs with recipients on presumed 'objective' grounds, such as tissue type, body size, time on waiting list, seriousness of need. However, even in this system, it is obvious that such a criterion as 'serious need' can be used in a manipulative way. Still, this system is preferable to the subjective use of criteria of social worth and status that would unfairly skew the distribution of organs.

Can allocation decisions be based on judgements about 'quality of life'?

Under conditions of scarcity, the question may arise in PCTs whether a patient's quality of life seems so poor that use of extensive medical inter-vention appears unwarranted. When this question is raised, it is important to consider who is making this quality of life judgement – the care team, the patient, or the patient's family? Several studies have shown that physi-cians often rate the patient's quality of life much lower than the patient does. When quality of life is considered unacceptable, an attempt should be made to make explicit the criteria that are being used in making that judgement. These criteria are often unspoken and can be influenced by bias or prejudice. A dialogue between carers and the patient can reveal some underlying concerns that may be addressed in other ways. Quality of life judgements based on prejudices against age, ethnicity, mental status, socio-economic status or sexual orientation are generally not relevant to considerations of diagnosis and treatment. Furthermore, they should not be used, explicitly or implicitly, by PCTs as the basis for rationing medical services.

What about 'macro-allocation' concerns?

Some situations involve what is often called 'macro-allocation', that is, broad policies to distribute resources across populations, as distinguished from 'micro-allocation' decisions, such as to give priority to one patient over another. Many of these reasons for shortage are the result of deliberate decisions to ration. Even such shortages as vital organs result from social policies that favour voluntary donation over routine salvaging of organs. The theoretical ethical question is: can a fair and just way of allocating healthcare resources be devised? The practical ethical question is: can a fair and just allocation be actually implemented in a particular social, economic and medical climate?

Ethical aspects of a 'right to healthcare'?

Several ethical theories have been elaborated to formulate criteria for fair and just distribution and to examine the arguments for a 'right to healthcare'. At present, little agreement exists on any of these issues. Ideally, all persons should have access to a 'decent minimum' of healthcare necessary to sustain life, prevent illness, relieve distress and disability, so that each person may enjoy his or her fair share of the normal opportunity range for individuals in his or her society.

An example of devising an allocation system that concentrated on the criteria of efficiency and cost-effectiveness was the so-called Oregon experiment in the United States. For Medicaid patients, a list of medical procedures, ranked in terms of their cost/benefit ratio, was constructed to determine the reimbursement policy. Even with such a system, ethical criteria must also be considered: what is to be done if life-saving and life-sustaining interventions rank low on cost-effectiveness? Is it ethical to omit the rescue of a person from death because their rescue by, say, bone marrow transplantation is less cost-effective than some preventive measures? How is cost-effectiveness to be applied to persons with shorter natural life expectancy, such as the elderly? The Oregon research literature offers a rich source of possible transferable learning for new PCTs (e.g. Honigsbaum *et al.* 1995; Meads 1997).

Envoi

The epigraph to this essay reflects our concern as to how an organisation such as a PCT can be a 'caring organisation'. We would posit this can only be possible if we begin to consider the functions of the organisation within an ethical framework. Such a framework implies the notion of a method which provides a 'normative pattern of recurrent and related operations yielding cumulative and progressive results' (Lonergan 1971). Some suggestions as to what should be the basis of the method are contained within the principles described above, which are not prescriptive but provide useful sign-posts for the New NHS organisations.

As primary and community care becomes more and more multi-disciplinary, disagreements may arise as different groups interpret how these ethical principles might be applied to their particular situation and to ways in which they might influence decision thinking. Those from clinical professions with an emphasis on providing care to individual patients have an ethical tradition that emphasises patient autonomy and commitment to the individual; those from a public health background tend to emphasise balancing the good of the individual against the good of the many; while managers and finance directors will have a tradition that reflects good business ethics. There might well be conflict between these groups and it should be recognised that these conflicts might become more frequent and more explicit in the context of managed primary care, for it is there all the activities these groupings represent converge in one organisational entity.

It will be a challenge within the context of the Third Way to our day-to-day decision thinking to reconcile these differing ethical stances and thus make our trusts truly caring and examples of good fiduciary practice. 'We should spend more of our decision making concentrating on what is important ... articulating and understanding our values and using these values to select meaningful decisions to ponder, to create better alternatives ... and to evaluate more carefully the desirability of the alternatives' (Keeney 1992). If PCTs behave accordingly, and trust in true experience, then they themselves will genuinely deserve to be taken on trust.

References

Beauchamp T and Childress J (1994) *Principles of Biomedical Ethics* (4e). Oxford University Press, New York.

Downie RS and Calnan KC (1994) *Healthy Respect: ethics in health care.* Oxford University Press, Oxford.

Honigsbaum F, Calltorp J, Ham C and Holstrom S (1995) *Priority Setting Processes for Healthcare.* Radcliffe Medical Press, Oxford.

Kass L (1985) *Towards a More Natural Science*. Free Press, New York.

Keeney RL (1992) *Value Focused Thinking*. Harvard University Press, Cambridge, MA.

Lindblom CE (1959) The science of muddling through. *Public Admin Rev.* **19**(3): 79–88.

Lonergan BJF (1971) *Method in Theology*. Darton, Longman & Todd, London.

March JG (1982) Theories of choice and making decisions. *Society.* **20**: 29–39.

Meads G (1997) The Oregon experience. In: B Sawyer and H Kogan (eds) *The Primary Healthcare Management Handbook*. Kogan Page, London. pp. 215–32.

Rawls J (1972) *A Theory of Justice*. Oxford University Press, Oxford.

Tudor Hart J (1988) *A New Kind of Doctor*. Merlin Press, London.

Central guidance

The following lists, in chronological order, the main sources of guidance from the Department of Health's published documentation on primary care trusts at the time of writing, with brief explanatory notes.

1 Health Service Circular 1998/228 (December 1998) *The New NHS: modern, dependable.*
   Primary Care Groups: delivering the agenda. NHSE, Leeds.
   Details for the first time the roles and responsibilities of the new primary care organisations in a single comprehensive form with pp. 100–103 setting the timetable for the introduction of primary care trusts.

2 Denham J (February 1999) *Primary Care Trusts.* Letter to NHS Chairs and Chief Executives. Department of Health, London.
   Clear ministerial direction and commitment given to the early development of PCTs with clarification of board membership and functions and future public accountabilities.

3 NHSE (December 1999) *Primary Care Trusts: establishment, the preparatory period and their functions.* Department of Health, London.
   Specific directions on powers delegated from health authorities to PCTs, governance requirements plus competency and role specifications for board members. The framework for 4 and 8 below.

4 NHSE (December 1999) *Working Together: human resources guidance and requirements for primary care trusts.* Department of Health, Leeds.
   Seeks to ensure PCTs (and their PMS initiatives) comply fully with NHS policies (e.g. equal opportunities) and standards (e.g. continuing professional development); covering staff transfers, clearing house arrangements, duty of partnerships and terms and conditions issues.

5 NHSE (December 1999) *Primary Care Trusts: financial framework.* Department of Health, Leeds.
   Very important document setting out statutory requirements of PCTs for financial accountability and control. Includes HCHS and GMS revenue and capital allocation arrangements, and is the basis for six

further documents to PCTs on such specifics as the PCT Manuals of Accounts, Capital Accounting and Costs, Prescribing Incentive Schemes and PCT Management Allowances. These were issued in January 2000.

6 NHSE (December 1999) *Primary Care Trusts: a guide to estate and facilities matters.* Department of Health, Leeds.
Covers PCTs' rights to own, transfer, share and dispose of property and requirements for inclusion in the Primary Care Investment Plan (PCIP).

7 Health Service Circular 1999/244 (December 1999) *Planning for Health and Health Care.* Department of Health, London.
Annually reviewed essential guidance which combines development and monitoring mechanisms and measures of the NHS as a whole, and what PCTs are expected to contribute to the HImP, SaFF, AAA and other vehicles for regulatory financial and activity information. Annex E tabulates the reporting requirements for all sections on NHS performance indicators for PCTs.

8 NHSE (February 2000) *IM&T Requirements to Support Primary Care Groups and Primary Care Trusts.* Department of Health, Leeds.
Translates new NHS Information Strategy information for health for PCTs and pulls together all relevant central guidance on requirements for data quality, commissioning, prescribing and performance management. Covers PCT business system requirements and foreshadows computerised clinical record systems.

9 Health Service Circular 2000/005 (March 2000) *Primary Care Trust and Group Allowances.* Department of Health, Leeds.
Reimbursement rules and rates for PCT Board, Executive and Sub-committee members and functions.

10 NHSE (April 2000) *Primary Care Trust HR Directory.* Department of Health, Wetherby.
Useful and periodically updated list of national and regional lead officers on a full range of PCT development issues.

11 Secretary of State for Health (July 2000) *The NHS Plan.* Department of Health, London.
The policy and resources agenda for the next decade with Chapters 6 and 7 most pertinent to PCTs as pooled budgets, unified commissioning and integrated providers pave the way for new Care Trusts.

12 Department of Health (December 2000) *NHS Plan Implementation Programme.* Department of Health, London.
Essential document for PCTs and other NHS organisations in converting new resource commitments into very specific but still incomplete

targets and timetables for service delivery and development; even at the level of numbers of new practice premises, location of resource centres etc.

Main contact point:

Richard Armstrong
Room 7E60
Health Services Directorate
NHS Executive
Department of Health
Quarry House
Quarry Hill
Leeds LS2 7UE
Tel: 0113 254 5191

Main local contacts:

Each health authority and regional office has a nominated PCT lead, and it is customary for PCTs to receive 'customised' versions of central documents according to their circumstances. The following is a typical illustration.

Local guidance – case example

1 *A PCT may be established by the Secretary of State following local consulta-tion, organised by the appropriate HA. Each PCT will be established as a free-standing NHS body separate from, but accountable to, its local HA. HAs will be required to delegate responsibility for commissioning the majority of hospital and community health services to PCTs. A level 4 PCT will also be able to provide services, run hospitals and community health services, and employ the necessary staff. HAs have a statutory duty to consult with the Local Medical Committee, and where these functions are delegated to a PCT, then the duty to consult the LMC will pass to the PCT as well.*

2 *Establishment, the preparatory period and functions guidance summary*
2.1 *The guidance sets out arrangements for establishing a PCT. It explains the key tasks which PCTs must undertake in their preparatory period and before the operational date. It outlines the functions of PCTs, including those functions that will be delegated and those where there is local flexibility for delegation.*
2.2 *The period between the establishment and operational dates is the preparatory period. During this period the PCT is limited in its range of functions to those required to prepare to become operational and the HA to which it is accountable*

will fund it. The CE is the Accountable Officer for the PCT and in each case (s)he will be appointed as such from the operational date of the PCT.

2.3 The Government's preferred PCT governance arrangements are set out in the guidance, including the respective roles of the PCT Board and Executive Committee. It sets out arrangements which should govern appointments, and makes clear that PCTs will have the same overall functions as PCGs and will be given responsibility for the provision of services across the broad mass of HA functions.

2.4 Appointments to PCTs should set a high standard by using the best HR practices, and candidates should be selected from clear job and person specifications after open and fair competition. PCTs will be major contributors to the delivery of national targets and service objectives and HAs will need to work closely with PCTs to ensure their full involvement in the local HImP. Each PCT should also prepare a PCIP that summarises their overall intentions for the development of primary care provision across its area. To facilitate the high quality service for patients, PCTs should seek the best possible co-terminosity with other bodies, in particular with the HA and LA. PCTs should consider a pooled budget with their local authority (LA) in order to facilitate partnership working and collaboration.

3 Guidance on issues surrounding employment policies and procedures

3.1 Staff who transfer into the PCT will bring with them a comprehensive package of terms and conditions of employment. There will, however, be no urgent need to harmonise most policies and procedures with one exception. It is important that disciplinary and grievance procedures are standardised in order to reflect the management arrangements in the new organisation and provide a level playing field for all staff. In relation to pay, PCTs, like other NHS organisations, are strongly advised to wait for the implementation of the new national pay system, which is currently under discussion.

4 Clinical governance and staff training and development

4.1 All staff will need to have access to suitable training opportunities. This will include a fair and objective method of identifying training needs, most likely through personal development plans (PDPs), linking with equal opportunities policies and be creating an organisational environment that will enable staff to be released for training and, where necessary provide cover in their absence. Influencing the Education Consortia at an early stage will support the workforce planning programme and ensure that the investment plans are able to develop the local health economy as a whole including primary care requirements. This will need to include smaller professional groups such as therapists as well as larger groups such as nurses and midwives. The PCT will also be responsible for locally managed systems of continuing professional development (CPD) as one of the cornerstones for implementing clinical governance.

A fair and objective appraisal system is the starting point for identifying the learning needs of individuals and teams. This will be further supported through the PDP process, which will reflect local service objectives, and clinical governance objectives as well as individual career aspirations.

5 Contractor status of general practitioners

5.1 GPs remain as independent self-employed GMS contractors providing specified services to the NHS. They will also retain the right to employ their own staff to support this service delivery. But PCTs will provide the opportunity for the sharing of good practices in all areas and this will include HR. Those staff who work in general practice but who are employed by NHS trusts will be unchanged in their employment status if their part of the organisation is not transferring to the PCT. Staff participation in PMS pilots was based on voluntary secondments rather than transfers of employment and there must be clear arrangements for secondees to return to their original NHS employer.

6 Composition of the PCT Board and Executive Committee

Committee	Membership
PCT Board	11 members Lay Chair (appointed by Secretary of State) 5 non-executive members (appointed by Secretary of State) Chief Executive Director of Finance 3 professional executive committee members including the EC Chair (a GP and a nurse)
PCT Executive Committee	up to 13 members Chair (chosen by professional members of the EC and ratified by the PCT Board) up to 10 professional members (a broad balance between GPs and other clinicians, but including nurses, other community professionals, public health expertise) Chief Executive Director of Finance Social Services Department representative

7 PCT property requirements

7.1 In each PCT's Establishment Order, the Secretary of State may impose restrictions on the exercise of functions by the PCT. It is envisaged that the main restrictions which will be applied are that they will not provide services directly to patients (level 3), or be limited to providing certain types of services, i.e. community health services (level 4).

7.2 *All PCTs need to prepare a PCIP. In managing their estate, they will be able to modernise, acquire and dispose of property. Any plans will need to be agreed with the HA in a PCIP that supports the HImP. The PCIP will also need to reflect plans to improve or modernise property owned or leased by general practitioners (GPs).*

7.3 *It should be recognised that the condition and fitness for purpose of some estate proposed for transfer to PCTs may not be to an ideal standard. Any proposals to bring such estate to the desired standard need to be included in the PCIP.*

7.4 *The PCIP should ensure that an appropriate estate is provided that is able to meet changing patterns of delivery or demand for services. While state provision supports the delivery of services, rather than driving it, it plays an important role in both modernising services and increasing the ability of the PCT to make changes to the way services are delivered.*

7.5 *PCTs should appoint a Board member to be responsible for health and safety (including fire safety).*

7.6 *The schedule of estate to be transferred to it on its establishment may comprise a range of accommodation including community hospitals, health centres, walk-in centres and clinics as well as office accommodation.*

Edited extract from *Consultation document*
for future PCT configuration options.
Camden and Islington Health Authority
July 2000

APPENDIX 2

Sources

Part 1 draws on individual semi-structured interviews during the June–August 2000 period with Chief Executives/Executive Directors from the following PCG/Ts:

Eastleigh
Marylebone
Middlesborough
North Islington
North Peterborough
Somerset Coast
South Croydon
Southampton East
Totton and Waterside
West Dorset

Parts 1 and 2 draw on development programmes and workshops facilitated by the Health Management Group and its associates with PCG/Ts across England between April 1998 and August 2000. Principal locations were:

Battersea
Bradford
Bromley
Camden
Croydon
East Hampshire
East Kent
East London and City
East Sussex
Enfield
Haringey
Hillingdon
Islington
Lambeth, Southwark and Lewisham
Leeds

Newcastle
North and East Devon
North Essex
North Hampshire
North Yorkshire
Nottingham
Oldham
Peterborough
Somerset
Southampton City
Southampton East
Totton and Waterside
Tower Hamlets
West Kent
Wolverhampton

For further details of individual studies please contact chapter contributors c/o Health Management Group, City University, Northampton Square, London EC1V 0HB.

Index